OBSTETRIC ANALGESIA AND ANESTHESIA

A Manual for Medical Students, Physicians in Training, Midwives, Nurses, and Other Health Personnel, Prepared for the World Federation of Societies of Anaesthesiologists

Second Edition, Revised

by
John J. Bonica, MD, DSc, FFARCS

Editorial Board

J. Selwyn Crawford, MB, ChB, FFARCS, FRCOG
Gertie Marx, MD
Sol M. Shnider, MD
Kevin McCaul, MD
John C. Hargrove, MD
David Ralston, MD
Toshio Akamatsu, MD
Fernando Rodriguez, MD

World Federation of
Societies of Anaesthesiologists
Amsterdam • 1980

JOHN J. BONICA, MD, DSc, FFARCS

Professor, Chairman Emeritus, Department of Anesthesiology,
Director, Pain Center, University of Washington School of Medicine,
Seattle, Washington, USA

WFSA Ad Hoc Committee for Obstetric Analgesia and Anesthesia

Chairman: John J. Bonica

Members: Ermelando V. Cosmi
             J. Selwyn Crawford
             Cenon Cruz
             Marcel M. Gemperle
             Harry Grant-Whyte
             Alvaro Guilherme Eugenio
             Jean Lassner
             Gertie Marx
             Kevin McCaul
             Nobuo Nishimura
             Fernando Rodriguez de la Fuente
             Michael Rosen
             Sol M. Shnider
             Emil A. Stojanov

International Standard Book Number: ISBN 0-9604882-0-0
Library of Congress Catalog Card Number: 80–53042

World Federation of Societies of Anaesthesiologists
% Department of Anesthesiology, RN–10
University of Washington School of Medicine
Seattle, WA 98195   USA

First Edition published 1972 by Springer-Verlag Berlin, Heidelberg

Printed in the United States of America

CONTENTS

PREFACE

The provision of the best anesthetic care to the greatest number of patients all over the world has always been the main goal of the World Federation of Societies of Anaesthesiologists (WSFA). In addition to the establishment of regional anesthesiology training centers, the organization of regional and world congresses, and the recent development of Visiting Educational Teams (VET), the distribution of practical monographs on some important aspects of anesthesiology has been considered important for the achievement of this objective. In 1971, WFSA President, Francis F. Foldes, after considering various areas of need, appointed an *Ad Hoc* Committee on Obstetric Analgesia-Anesthesia charged with the task of compiling a brief but comprehensive monograph on obstetric analgesia and anesthesia and infant resuscitation. Dr. Foldes was prompted to take this action by the following considerations: (a) in most countries throughout the world, a significant number of paturients receive analgesia-anesthesia; (b) in most countries, the majority of obstetric anesthetics are relegated to medical and paramedical personnel untrained in the administration of the potent drugs and techniques used for obstetric pain relief, with consequent preventable maternal and perinatal morbidity and even mortality; and (c), since most vaginal and abdominal deliveries require "emergency anesthesia" and since two lives are at stake, the parturient deserves expert anesthetic care.

The chairman of the *Ad Hoc* Committee, with the help of several of its members, developed the first edition of this monograph in time for the Vth World Congress held in Kyoto in September, 1972. The monograph was received very favorably and subsequently, over 26,000 copies of the English version were distributed throughout the world. The monograph was also translated and published in French, Turkish, and Spanish.

The gratifying response to the first edition undoubtedly reflected the impressive surge of interest in this field that has occurred during the past decade or so. This trend has exerted and today continues to exert pressure on physicians, midwives, and obstetric nurses to provide parturients with better, more widespread pain relief during childbirth. Of the many factors of this trend for greater demand for, and use of, analgesia-anesthesia for childbirth, one of the most important has been the expectation of parturients. During the past decade or so, gravidas in many countries, having been made aware of the benefits of good obstetric analgesia by magazine articles, books, television, and news media, have come to expect it, just as they expect painless surgery and painless dentistry. This increased demand by patients and the realization that lack of anesthesia and poorly administered anesthesia in themselves cause maternal and perinatal morbidity and mortality have prompted obstetricians in many parts of the world to demand better services by anesthetists. This expectation is strongly supported by statistics from those medical centers where obstetric analgesia-anesthesia is provided by competent personnel. These data show that optimal pain relief not only does *not* contribute to, but also actually reduces maternal and perinatal morbidity and mortality by permitting better obstetric care.

This second edition, as the first, is intended to provide a concise overview and guidelines to medical students; physicians in anesthesia, obstetric, and pediatric training programs; obstetricians; obstetric nurses; midwives; and others interested in this field. Although, since the first edition, eight books on this subject have been published in English (and possibly some in other languages), these are usually too detailed, too long, and too expensive for the aforementioned groups. On the other hand, the overviews of the most important aspects of this subject are sufficiently comprehensive to be useful to anyone who is not an expert obstetric anesthetist.

The advent of a significant amount of new information since the appearance of the first edition of this monograph has made it necessary to rewrite much of the text and develop more illustrations summarizing physiologic, physiopathologic, and pharmacologic facts and depicting techniques of regional analgesia-anesthesia. The importance of fundamental knowledge in managing parturients cannot be overemphasized and is attested to by the large amount of space devoted to its concern in Part A. Since normal vaginal delivery occurs in over three-quarters of births, a commensurate amount of space is devoted to this aspect of obstetrics. It deserves emphasis that many regional anesthetic techniques and general anesthesia, though apparently deceptively simple, require not only knowledge but the acquisition of skill and experience under the supervision of an expert obstetric anesthetist. The sections on anesthesia in the presence of complications and for operative deliveries consider only the most common problems. The scope of the brochure and space limitations preclude discussion of every drug and technique used throughout the world or a detailed review of the literature of the methods mentioned. The reference list at the end of the monograph should be consulted for comprehensive reviews.

I wish to express sincere thanks and appreciation to the following persons for their valuable suggestions in the development of this second edition: Drs. J. Selwyn Crawford, Gertie Marx, Sol M. Shnider, Kevin McCaul, and F. Fernando Rodriquez de la Fuente, all of whom are members of the *Ad Hoc* Committee, and to Drs. David H. Ralston, John C. Hargrove, and Toshio Akamatsu, my colleagues in the Department of Anesthesiology, University of Washington School of Medicine. I also wish to thank my secretaries, Monica Zucker and Dorothy Burger, for their help in the preparation of the manuscript; Marjorie Domenowske for the development of a number of the illustrations; and Louisa Jones for invaluable expertise in editing and proofreading the manuscript. Arthur Catalani, President of Breon Laboratories USA, deserves special thanks and appreciation for providing significant support for the project. Finally, I also wish to thank the authors and publishers of the books and articles from which a number of illustrations and tables have been borrowed or modified.

John J. Bonica, MD, DSc, FFARCS
Seattle, Washington USA
July 1, 1980

PART A.   FUNDAMENTAL CONSIDERATIONS

To provide optimal obstetric anesthetic care, it is essential for the anesthetist* to know well the maternal physiologic alterations produced by pregnancy, labor, and parturition; physiology and pharmacology of the fetal placental complex and of the forces of labor; and how these are altered by analgesics and anesthetics. Unless this knowledge is properly applied, the anesthetist may make a grievous error that may prove disastrous to the mother or the newborn or both. A summary of the current knowledge of the maternal physiologic and psychologic changes produced by pregnancy and parturition will be given in Chapter 1; a summary of the physiology and pharmacology of the placenta, fetus, and newborn is given in Chapter 2; and the physiology and pharmacology of the forces of labor and the pain of parturition are discussed in Chapter 3.

CHAPTER 1.   MATERNAL PHYSIOLOGIC AND PSYCHOLOGIC ALTERATIONS

The process of pregnancy, labor, and delivery produces remarkable physiologic changes in the mother, and these and anesthesia will have important impacts on the gravida. From the viewpoint of optimal anesthetic care, the changes involving circulation, respiration, acid-base and electrolyte balance, and the gastrointestinal, renal, and hepatic functions are the most important. These changes, produced by placental hormones or due to mechanical effects of the growing uterus or both, develop to meet the increasing metabolic needs of the maternal-fetal-placental complex. They also prepare the gravida for the stresses of parturition and the subsequent occlusion of the placental circulation.

CIRCULATORY CHANGES

The Blood

Blood Volumes. Beginning at 6–8 weeks of pregnancy, there is a progressive increase in total blood, plasma, and red cell volumes which reach maximum at 28–32 weeks and then remain constant until parturition. Although there is marked variation among gravidas, the "average" values are listed in Table 1 and depicted in Figure 1. The hypervolemia of pregnancy is accommodated by the

---

* Throughout this volume the term, anesthetist, will be used to denote the person who administers the anesthetic, whether a trained physician (anesthetist), certified nurse anesthetist (CNA), or other allied health personnel.

enlarged uterus and breasts and the increased blood flow to kidneys, skeletal muscles, and skin and parallels the increased cardiac output and ventilation. These changes facilitate maternal/fetal exchange of blood gases, nutrients, and metabolites and enable the gravida to tolerate the normal blood loss during parturition. The measured loss is 300–500 ml with vaginal delivery and 600–1,000 ml with abdominal (cesarean) delivery. By 8 weeks postpartum, the blood volume and its constituents have returned to nonpregnant values. (See Figures 1 and 2.)

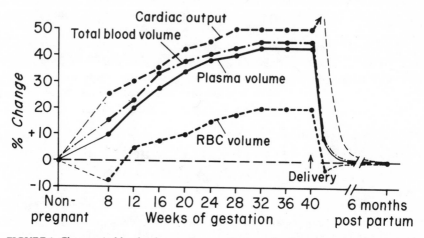

FIGURE 1. Changes in blood volume, plasma volume, red cell volume, and cardiac output during pregnancy and in the puerperium. The curves were constructed from various reports in the literature and illustrate trends in percent change rather than absolute values.

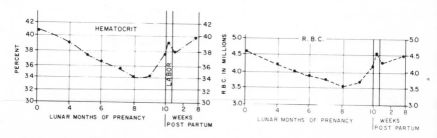

FIGURE 2. Hemoglobin and hematocrit values during pregnancy and the puerperium.

Blood Composition. The greater increase in plasma volume (50%) than the increase in red cell mass (30%) results in hemodilution with consequent decrease in red cell count, hemoglobin, and hematocrit—the so-called "physiologic anemia" of pregnancy. Proper nutrition and iron and folic acid supplementation will lessen the magnitude of these changes, and the healthy gravida is able to maintain these blood components above the accepted minimums of 3.5 million RBC, 11 grams hemoglobin, and 35% hematocrit. Values below these reflect iron deficiency anemia and require active therapy.

TABLE 1. CHANGES IN BLOOD AND ITS CONSTITUENTS DURING PREGNANCY

VARIABLE	NONPREGNANT	AVERAGE VALUES MAXIMUM DURING PREGNANCY	CHANGE
A. Volumes (ml)			
Total blood	4,000	5,700	+40%
Plasma	2,700	4,000	+50%
Red cell	1,300	1,700	+30%
B. Formed Elements			
RBC (million/μl)	4.6	3.6	−1.0
Hemoglobin (gm %)	14	12	−2.0
Hematocrit (%)	41	35	−6.0
WBC	6,000	9,000	+3,000
Platelets	200,000 − 300,000	same	no change
C. Total Proteins			
Amount (gm)	290	350	↑
Concentration (gm/100 ml)	7.3	6.5	↓
D. Albumin			
Total (gm)	127	144	↑
Concentration (gm/100 ml)	5.5	4.4	↓
E. Total Globulins	Slight relative and absolute increase		
Alpha	Slight increase		
Beta	Slight increase		
Gamma	Slight increase		
F. Electrolytes (mEq/L)			
Total Base	155	143	↓
Na^+	143	138	↓
K^+	4.3	4.1	↓
Ca^+	4.8	4.6	↓
Total Anions			
HCO^3	25	23	↓
G. Blood Gases and Acid-Base			
PaO_2 (mm Hg)	95	105	↑
$PaCO_2$ (mm Hg)	40	32	↓
Buffer base (mEq/L)	47	42	↓
Base excess (mEq/L)	0.0	−3.0	↓
pH	7.4	7.4 − 7.42	no change or slight ↑

There is also an increase in total circulating proteins, but, because of the hemodilution, the concentration of the total proteins and the albumin fraction decrease, as do the specific gravity and viscosity of the blood. Since there is a concommitant relative as well as absolute increase in total globulins (with variation of different fractions—see Table 1), the albumin–globulin ratio declines but is not reversed. There is also a significant increase in fibrinogen, which, together with the increase in plasma globulins, causes a progressive and marked increase in the erythrocyte sedimentation rate. Moreover, there is an increase in certain components of the coagulation process (factors I, VII, VIII, IX, and X) and a progressive increase in the serum, fibrin-fibrinogen degradation factor. Although these suggest that both fibrin formation and fibrinolysis increase as pregnancy progresses, gestation is associated with a hypercoagulable state that constitutes a double-edged sword: it protects the gravida against excessive blood loss during parturition but also increases the risk of thromboembolism.

Other changes in the constituency of the blood are listed in Table 1. The oxygen and carbon dioxide dissociation curves of maternal blood are shifted to the right, while those of the fetal blood are shifted to the left. During pregnancy the serum cholinesterase activity decreases about 20–30%, but the enzyme remains qualitatively unchanged, and the decreased amount is sufficient for normal hydrolysis of succinylcholine, chloroprocaine, and other drugs degraded by plasma.

Hemodynamic Changes during Pregnancy

Cardiac Output. Early in the first trimester, cardiac output begins a progressive increase that reaches a maximum of 40–50% above normal at 28–32 weeks and then continues at these levels until parturition. The increase is the product of both an increase in heart rate of 10–15 beats per minute and a 30% increase in stroke volume. Figure 3 depicts the marked differences in these three variables, measured in the lateral and supine positions, especially during the last trimester, when the enlarged uterus compresses the inferior vena cava and other veins at the pelvic brim. This venous compressing effect is greatest in the supine position, significantly less in the lateral position, and least in the knee-chest position.

Blood Pressures. Arterial blood pressure decreases slightly during pregnancy because of the concommitant 20–25% decrease in total peripheral resistance which more than offsets the increase in cardiac output (Figure 4). Since the diastolic pressure decreases more than the systolic, the decrease in mean arterial pressure is greater than the decrease in systolic pressure, and the pulse pressure is increased. Central and forearm venous pressures remain normal, but the femoral venous pressure increases progressively as pregnancy advances, and the uterus continues to enlarge and compress the inferior vena cava (and the aorta). This is compensated in part by the diversion of blood through the internal vertebral venous plexus and thence through the azygos venous system which empties into the superior vena cava.

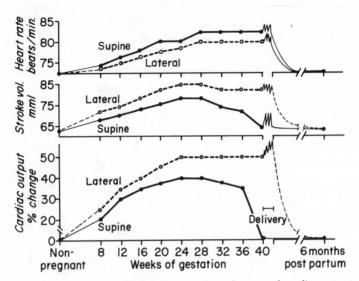

FIGURE 3. Changes in maternal heart rate, stroke volume, and cardiac output during pregnancy with the gavida in the supine position and in the lateral position. These curves are based on data derived from several studies, including Ueland, K., et al.: Am. J. Obstet. Gynecol. 104:856, 1969.

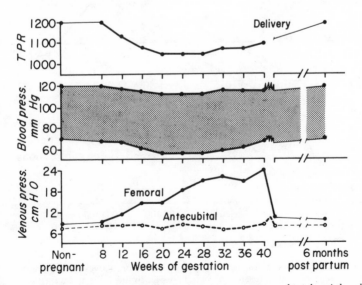

FIGURE 4. Changes in arterial blood pressure, venous pressure, and total peripheral resistance during pregnancy.

5

Other Changes. The cephalad displacement of the diaphragm by the enlarging uterus causes the heart to be shifted to the left and anteriorily and produces functional changes including louder heart sounds with an accentuated first apical and second pulmonic sound, a faint hemic systolic murmur over pulmonary and tricuspic areas, and a more forceful, palpable apical beat. The electrocardiogram may show a large Q wave and an inverted T wave in leads III, V_1 and V_2, a progressive tendency toward left axis deviation from the second to sixth month, and, occasionally, depression of S-T segment and flattening of T wave. All of these ECG changes disappear during the puerperium.

Hemodynamics during Parturition

During labor *cardiac output* increases above prelabor. Between contractions, cardiac output during the early first stage is about 15% above that of prelabor, during the late first stage it is about 30%, during the second stage about 45%, immediately after delivery it is 65% above prelabor, and one hour later it is 30–50% above prelabor. With each uterine contraction, the uterus is raised by action of the uterine ligaments and about 300–500 ml of blood is also squeezed out of the uterus into the central circulation. Consequently, stroke volume,

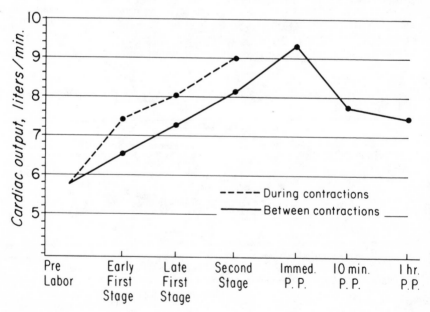

FIGURE 5. Cardiac output during various phases of labor, between contractions and during contractions. Note progressive increase between contractions and a further 15–20 percent increase during contractions. (Developed from data of Hansen, J.M., and Ueland K., Acta Anaesthesiol. Scand. Suppl. 23:49, 1966.)

cardiac output, and left ventricular work increase. Each contraction consistently increases cardiac output 15–25% above that between contractions (Figure 5).

 Blood pressure, central venous pressure, and femoral venous pressure also increase with each uterine contraction. Arterial blood pressure increases 15–25 mm Hg systolic and 10–15 mm Hg diastolic (Figure 6). The magnitude of these changes varies and depends on the intensity of contractions and the associated pain, anxiety and apprehension, and the position of the parturient (see below). During the second stage, the bearing-down efforts often alter blood pressure in a way similar to the Valsalva's maneuver. The changes in venous pressure are rapidly transmitted to the internal vertebral venous plexus, and thus cause a transient rise in extradural and cerebrospinal fluid pressure (Figure 6). These changes are greater in the supine than in the lateral position.

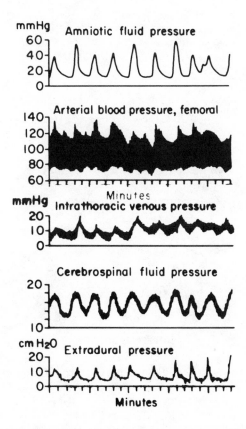

FIGURE 6. Hemodynamic effects of uterine contractions. Note the increase in arterial blood pressure and central venous pressure which is reflected in cerebrospinal fluid and extradural pressures.

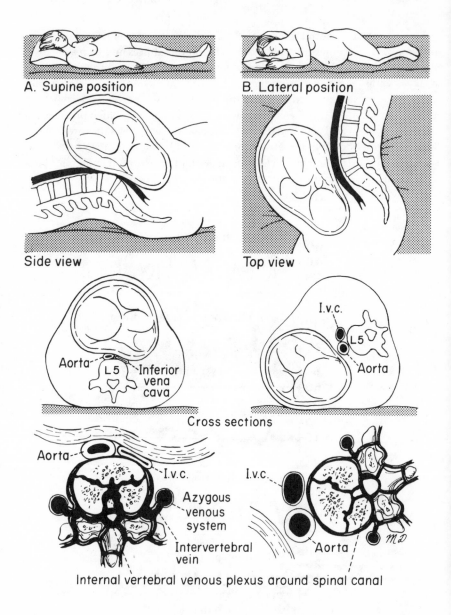

A. Supine position

B. Lateral position

Side view

Top view

Aorta · L5 · Inferior vena cava

I.v.c. · L5 · Aorta

Cross sections

Aorta · I.v.c. · Azygous venous system · Intervertebral vein

I.v.c. · Aorta

Internal vertebral venous plexus around spinal canal

FIGURE 7. The effects of the pregnant uterus on the inferior vena cava and the aorta in the supine position (left) and the lateral position (right). The marked aortocaval compression in the supine position causes venous blood to be diverted to and through the vertebral venous plexus which becomes very engorged, thus reducing the size of the epidural and subarachnoid spaces.

Aortocaval Compression

The compression of the inferior vena cava and the lower aorta at the pelvic brim caused by the enlarged uterus produces marked hemodynamic changes, particularly when the gravida assumes the supine position (Figures 7, 8). The obstruction of the inferior vena cava and the pelvic veins reduces the venous return to the heart and consequently the cardiac output. The venous obstruction is usually offset by two compensatory mechanisms: (1) increase in sympathetic tone with generalized vasoconstriction, increase in total peripheral resistance and heart rate, and (2) diversion of some of the blood through the internal verte-bral venous plexus. In 90% of gravidas, these compensatory mechanisms are sufficiently effective to maintain the arterial blood pressure at near normal levels. However, in the other 10% of gravidas, the obstruction is so great and the amount of blood returned to the heart and the consequent cardiac output are so low that despite the intense vasoconstriction and tachycardia, blood pressure

SITES OF OBSTRUCTION

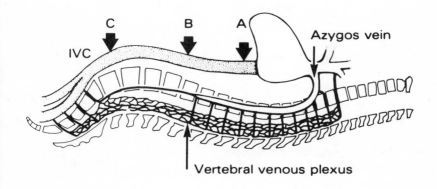

FIGURE 8. Diagram of the caval venous system and its connections with the vertebral and azygous systems. Commonest sites of compression of the inferior vena cava (IVC) are: (a) suprahepatic in lordotic position; (b) uterus at term; and (c) pressure at pelvic brim in exaggerated lordosis and term pregnancy. (Courtesy of Bromage, P. R., *Epidural Analgesia:* Philadelphia, W. B. Saunders, 1978.)

falls precipitously, causing the so-called *supine hypotensive syndrome* (Figure 9). In severe cases, this syndrome becomes evident within seconds, but, in moderate cases, hypotension does not develop for 3–5 minutes after the patient has assumed the supine position. This condition can begin to develop during the second trimester, becomes maximal at 36–38 weeks, and may decrease with the descent of the fetal head into the pelvis.

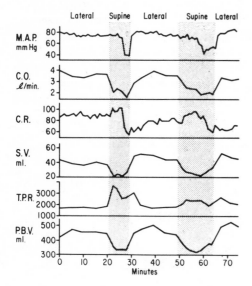

FIGURE 9. The profound influence of the supine position on maternal hemodynamics in a parturient with the supine hypotensive syndrome. The impairment of venous return consequent to the pressure of the gravid uterus markedly decreased stroke volume (SV) and cardiac rate (CR), and consequently cardiac output (CO), and also reduced pulmonary blood volume (PBV). The compensatory increase in cardiac rate (CR) and total peripheral resistance (TPR) maintained blood pressure for about 5 minutes, but then the patient developed a marked reduction in mean arterial pressure (MAP). (Modified from and courtesy of Scott, D. B., Br. J. Anaesth. 40:120–128, 1968.)

The compression of the lower aorta leads to decreased blood flow to the kidneys, uterus, and lower extremities. As a result, maternal urine output and kidney function are significantly lower in the supine as compared with the lateral position, and fetal arrhythmia, indicative of fetal-placental insufficiency, may develop soon after the mother assumes a supine position. They are relieved when she changes to the lateral position. In contrast to the caval compression, there is no compensation for the effects of the aortic compression, However, both are preventable by uterine displacement achieved manually or left down tilt and wedge under the right buttock.

During labor, the compressive phenomena in the supine position are exaggerated by uterine contractions (Figure 10). As the uterus tenses and hardens and increases its pressure on the major veins and arteries across the pelvic brim, there is often an apparent improvement in the mother's circulation but a hidden deterioration of the fetal environment. Each contraction tips the uterus around a fulcrum formed by the lumbosacral vertebral prominence, and aortic compression is increased, leading to a hyperdynamic circulation above the compression but a further deterioration below it. Consequently, there is a steep rise of mater-

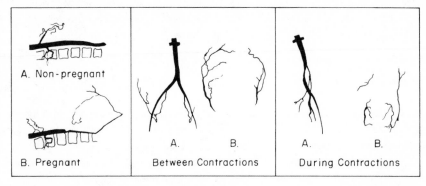

FIGURE 10. Effects of the enlarged uterus and uterine contractions on the aorta and placental circulation. *Left panel* shows the outline of the abdominal aorta and its branches in the nonpregnant state (a) and the pregnant state (b). *Middle panel* depicts the outline of the lower aorta, iliac arteries, and uterine arteries (a) and an adequate perfusion of the placenta (b). *Right panel* shows that during contractions the uterus compresses the lower portion of the aorta and obliterates the right iliac and uterine arteries (a) and markedly diminishes placental perfusion (b). (Modified from and courtesy of Bieniarz, J., et al. Am. J. Obstet. Gynecol. 100:203, 1978.)

nal cardiac output and a hypertensive rise of blood pressure above the obstruction but a fall below, as depicted in Figure 11). Figure 10 depicts the degree of aortic compression that can occur during uterine contraction in the supine posi-

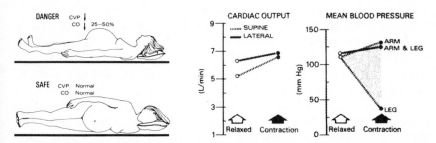

FIGURE 11. Cardiovascular effects of posture and uterine contractions. The *left panel* shows the hazards of supine position which causes a decrease in central venous pressure and cardiac output, but these promptly return to normal when the parturient assumes the lateral position. The *right panel* shows the changes in cardiac output and blood pressure during and between contractions. During contractions in the supine position, the cardiac output increases and pressure rises in the upper limb but falls in the lower limb, because of partial aortic obstruction during uterine contractions. This effect is avoided by placing the parturient in the lateral position, which facilitates return of blood from the lower limbs to the general circulation so that cardiac output and blood pressure are maintained at a high resting level between contractions. Consequently, during contractions, the increase in cardiac output and blood pressure is less than in the supine position. (Courtesy of Bromage, P.R.; *Epidural Analgesia*, Philadelphia, W.B. Saunders, 1978. Constructed from data of Ueland and Hansen, 1969, Galbert and Marx, 1974, and Bieniarz et al, 1968.)

tion. Moreover, almost the entire 300–500 ml of blood squeezed out of the uterus is forced into the extradural and azygous systems during contractions, causing heightened peaks of extradural venous pressure.

Clinical Implications

The aforementioned changes in blood volume, blood constituency, and hemo-dynamics produced by pregnancy, parturition, and the puerperium are of great relevance to anesthetic care. The increase in blood volume increases cardiac pre-load, but this is compensated for by the significant reduction in the afterload consequent to the reduction of total peripheral resistance and blood viscocity. Although this hyperdynamic state increases cardiac workload and predisposes the development of functional murmurs, healthy gravidas have no impairment in cardiac reserve, as attested in part by the fact that cardiac output during exer-cise remains within the usual range. On the other hand, in gravidas with heart disease and consequent low myocardial reserve, the increase in work of the heart may constitute too great a strain and may precipitate pulmonary conges-tion. In such patients it is especially important to obviate further increase in the work of the heart during labor by providing effective analgesia, preferably with regional techniques.

The diversion of blood consequent to the venous compression causes the in-ternal vertebral venous plexus to become greatly engorged, and the capillary cir-culation in the meninges is slowed. These changes make it necessary to reduce the volume and amount of local anesthetic to achieve subarachnoid or epidural block to at least 2/3 of those used for nonpregnant women. The reduced need for local anesthetics is present regardless of the position of the gravida and despite the immediate effect of left uterine displacement. Moreover, the slowed capillary meningeal circulation delays the absorption of these drugs into the blood, leav-ing more for the target nerves, and thus decreases the latency (time of onset) and increases the duration of analgesia.

The fluctuation in cerebrospinal fluid pressure produced by uterine contrac-tions, bearing-down efforts, or by straining, promotes turbulent currents in the fluid compartment. Consequently, injection of a local anesthetic into the subar-achnoid space during such conditions may result in abnormally high spinal an-esthesia. This may be accentuated by the exaggerated lumbar lordosis of preg-nant women.

The postural hemodynamic changes make it mandatory that gravidas avoid the supine position during the latter phases of pregnancy and during labor. Moreover, since induction of spinal or extradural anesthesia or other procedures that entail vasomotor blockade deprive gravidas of a compensatory vasoconstric-tion, they are likely to incur much greater falls in arterial blood pressure than nonpregnant patients. Unless prophylactic measures are carried out such severe hypotension may develop as to threaten the life of the mother and fetus. Prophylactic measures include infusion of fluids prior to the block, having the parturient on her side during the duration of anesthesia and labor, and effective lateral displacement of the uterus during the delivery. Unilateral predominance of the block can be avoided by having the patient change sides every 2–3 minutes during the induction period. It is aso desirable to ascertain the degree of compression and consequent supine hypotension prior to the induction of a block by measuring the blood pressure with the patient on the side and again at 2, 4, and 6 minutes after the patient has been in a supine position. This will permit diagnosis of supine hypotension in those gravidas who have delayed onset of the condition.

During the immediate postpartum period when the greatest increase in cardiac output occurs, the patient is able to maintain normal blood pressure by compensatory vasodilation. If the obstetric team deprives the mother of this compensatory vasodilation by administering an oxytocic with vasoconstrictor action such as ergonovine maleate (Ergotrate) and/or a potent peripheral vasopressor such as methoxamine (Vasoxyl) or phenylephrine (Neosynephrine), severe hypertension may develop which, in some patients, may cause a cerebrovascular accident. For this reason, it is preferable to use oxytocin and ephedrine to increase uterine contractility and blood pressure, respectively, during the delivery.

RESPIRATION

Pregnancy produces impressive anatomic and physiologic changes involving the patient's airway, lung volumes, ventilation, and the dynamics of breathing.

Anatomic Changes

In the majority of pregnant women, capillary engorgement takes place throughout the respiratory tract so that the nasopharynx, larynx, trachea, and bronchi become swollen and reddened. These changes simulate inflammation and often cause changes in the voice and make nose breathing difficult for some women at term. They are markedly aggravated in the presence of even minor upper respiratory infection and toxemia of pregnancy. The growing uterus causes the diaphragm to rise 4 cm but does not impair its excursions and, in fact, this is greater in pregnancy than in the puerperium. the abdominal muscles have much less tone and are less active in the pregnant than in the nonpregnant state. The cephalad displacement of the diaphragm is effectively counterbalanced by an increase of 2 cm in the anterior-posterior and transverse diameters of the thoracic cage and flaring of the ribs, all resulting in a 5–7 cm increase in the circumference of the thoracic cage (Figure 12). X-rays show increased lung markings that simulate mild congestive failure.

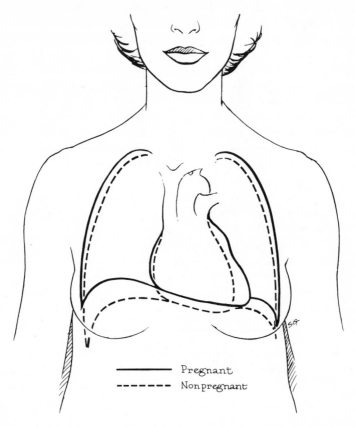

FIGURE 12. Changes in the outline of the heart, lungs, and thoracic cage that occur in pregnancy. The gradual migration of the uterus cephalad causes the diaphragm to move upward and thus encroach on the lungs, and causes the heart to be displaced laterally and anteriorally, but this is counterbalanced by an increase in the anterior-posterior and transverse diameters of the chest wall. (From Bonica, J.J.: *Principles and Practice of Obstetric Analgesia and Anesthesia*, Philadelphia, F. A. Davis Company, 1967, as modified from and courtesy of Klaften, E. and Palugyay, H: Arch.Gynaek. 78:1, 1959.)

Lung Volumes

Lung volumes do not change until the fifth month of gestation (Figures 13, 14), after which there is a progressive decrease in *expiratory reserve volume* (ERV), *residual volume* (RV), and *functional residual capacity* (FRC). At term, ERV is about 100–150 ml less, and RV 200 ml less than in the nonpregnant state. Consequently FRC is about 300–350 ml or 20% lower than in the nonpregnant state.

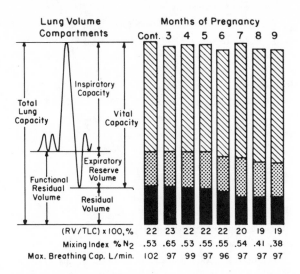

FIGURE 13. Serial measurements of lung volume compartments, pulmonary mixing index, and maximum breathing capacity during normal pregnancy. Control values were obtained from the same women 4–9 months postpartum. The mean values were obtained in 9 subjects by Cugell et al. (Am.Rev.Tubercul. 67:568, 1953). Note that changes begin after the 5th month. (Modified from and courtesy of Prowse, C.M., and Gaensler,, E.A., Anesthesiology 26:381, 1965.)

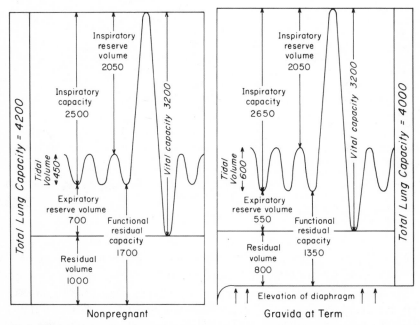

FIGURE 14. Pulmonary volumes and capacities in the nonpregnant state and in the gravida at term. (Courtesy of Bonica, J.J.: *Principles and Practice of Obstetric Analgesia and Anesthesia*, Philadelphia, F.A. Davis Company, 1967.)

15

These changes are accentuated by the recumbent position, obesity, and mitral valve disease. The *inspiratory capacity* (IC) increases 5%, but the *inspiratory reserve volume* (IRV) remains the same with the result that *total lung capacity* (TLC) decreases slightly (5%). *Vital capacity* (VC) remains unaltered, but occasionally increases (Table 2).

Closing capacity is unchanged during pregnancy, but the difference between closing capacity and functional residual capacity may be reduced, particularly in the supine position. This may result in lowered V_a/Q ratios in the dependent portions of the lung and may account for the lowered arterial PaO_2 in some parturients at term. *Airway resistance* is decreased, probably because of progesterone-induced relaxation of bronchial muscles, but *maximum breathing capacity* (MBC), *timed vital capcity*, and *diffusing capacity* remain unchanged. *Lung compliance* is also relatively unaffected, but *chest wall compliance* and thus total respiratory compliance are significantly decreased in late pregnancy, more so in the lithotomy than in the supine positions, but these rapidly increase after delivery of the infant. The mixing and distribution of inspired gas in the lung of the gravida remains normal.

TABLE 2.   CHANGES IN THE RESPIRATORY SYSTEM

VARIABLE	"AVERAGE" CHANGE	VARIABLE	"AVERAGE" CHANGE
Minute ventilation	↑ 50%	Residual volume	↓ 20%
Alveolar ventilation	↑ 70%	Functional residual capacity	↓ 20%
Tidal volume	↑ 40%		
Respiratory rate	↑ 15%	Inspiratory lung capacity	↑ 5%
Dead space	No change	Inspiratory reserve volume	No change
Airway resistance	↓ 36%	Vital capacity	No change
Total pulmonary resistance	↓ 50%	Total lung capacity	↓ 5%
Lung compliance (alone)	No change	Maximum breathing capacity	No change
Chest wall compliance (alone)	↓ 45%	Timed vital capacities	No change
Oxygen consumption	↑ 20%	Closing volume	No change or ↓
Expiratory reserve volume	↓ 20%		

Ventilation during Pregnancy

Pregnancy is associated with a marked increase in minute ventilation which at term is 50% above normal. This is effected by a 40% increase in tidal volume and a 15% increase in respiratory rate (Figure 15). Since dead space remains normal, alveolar ventilation is about 70% above normal at term. Earlier studies suggested that the increase was progressive throughout the pregnancy, but more recent data show that almost maximum hyperventilation occurs as early as the second or third month of gestation (Figure 16). The changes in lung volumes and ventilation lead to a reduction of arterial and alveolar carbon dioxide which averages 32 mm Hg at term, and a increase in the oxygen tension to about 105 mm Hg.

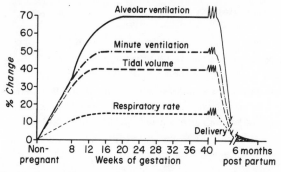

FIGURE 15. Changes in ventilatory parameters during pregnancy. Note that almost maximum hyperventilation occurs as early as the 2nd or 3rd month of gestation. Since the respiratory rate increases to a much lesser extent than tidal volume and dead space remains normal, the percent increase in alveolar ventilation is greater than the percent increase in minute ventilation. (Curves derived from data published by Bonica J.J.: *in Parturition and Perinatology*, Marx, G.F. (ed), Philadelphia, F.A. Davis, 1972; Enderson, G.J., et al., J. Obstet. Gynaecol. Br. Cwlth. 76:16, 1969; and Blechner, J.N., et al. Am. J. Obstet. Gynecol. 100:1, 1968.)

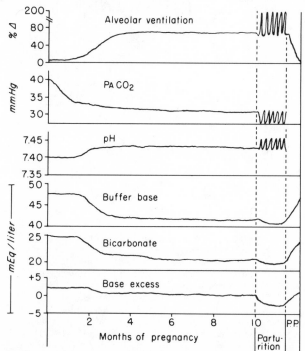

FIGURE 16. Alveolar ventilation, arterial carbon dioxide, pH, and acid-base changes during pregnancy, parturition, and postpartum period. With the nearly 80% increase in alveolar ventilation, the $PaCO_2$ decreases to levels of 32 mm Hg at term with concommitant changes in the acid-base. During parturition, further changes occur, especially during uterine contractions, that increase ventilation and decrease $PaCO_2$. All of these variables return to normal 1-3 weeks after delivery. (Courtesy of Bonica, J.J.: Clinical Anesthesia Series, Philadelphia, F.A. Davis Company, 10-2:9, 1973.)

Ventilation during Parturition

During parturition, ventilation is further increased by the pain of labor, anxiety and apprehension, or voluntarily in patients trained in natural childbirth or in psychoprophylaxis. The magnitude of hyperventilation varies greatly, depending on the circumstances: respiratory rates as high as 60–70 per minute, tidal volumes of up to 2250 ml, and maximum peak inspiratory flow rates of up to 340 L per minute have been reported. In untrained and unmedicated primiparas, minute ventilation increases from a normal of about 9 L per minute be-

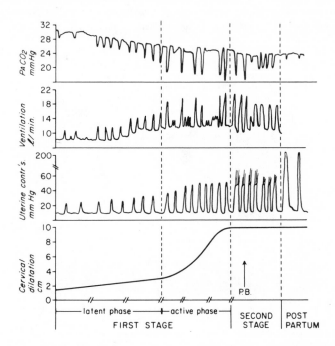

FIGURE 17. Ventilatory changes during labor in unpremedicated gravida (schematic). Note correlation of the stage of labor as reflected by the Friedman's curve (lowermost tracing), the frequency and intensity of uterine contractions, minute ventilation, and arterial carbon dioxide tension (uppermost curve). Early in labor, uterine contractions are small and are associated with mild pain, causing only small increases in minute ventilation and decreases in $PaCO_2$. But, as labor progresses, the greater intensity of contractions causes greater changes in ventilation and CO_2. During the active phase, contractions with increased intrauterine pressure of 40–60 mm Hg cause severe pain which acts as intense stimulus to ventilation with a consequent reduction of $PaCO_2$ to 18–20 mm Hg. During the second stage, the reflex bearing-down efforts further increase intrauterine pressure and distend the perineum with consequent additional pain that prompts the parturient to ventilate at a rate almost twice that of early labor, causing a commensurate reduction in $PaCO_2$. Pudendal block relieves the perineal pain, but the patient is still able to effectively bear down voluntarily. The voluntary bearing-down efforts decrease the respiratory rate and consequently minute volume ventilation, resulting in a smaller reduction in $PaCO_2$ than obtained before the block. (Courtesy of Bonica, J.J.: Clinical Anesthesia Series, Philadelphia, F.A. Davis Company, 10-2:9, 1973.)

tween contractions to 20–25 L and even as high as 35 L or more during peak of contractions. Consequently, the $PaCO_2$ falls to 20 mm Hg and some as low as 10–15 mm Hg, PaO_2 increases to 105–108 mm Hg, and pH increases to 7.5 and as high as 7.6 during the peak of contractions. During the second stage, parturients without adequate analgesia hyperventilate to an even greater extent during contractions between bouts of involuntary bearing-down efforts (Figure 17). As soon as the relaxation phase begins and pain no longer stimulates respiration, the hypocapnea causes a transient period of hypoventilation that may cause decrease in PaO_2 to hypoxic levels. The recent application of transcutaneous oxygen electrodes has shown that in parturients breathing air, the pain-induced hyperventilation and slight hyperoxia is followed by a transient period of hypoventilation and a decrease in arterial oxygen tension ranging from 5–50%, with a mean of 20%. When PaO_2 falls below 70 mm Hg, it has significant repercussions on the fetus consisting of lowering PaO_2 and late decelerations (Figure 18a).

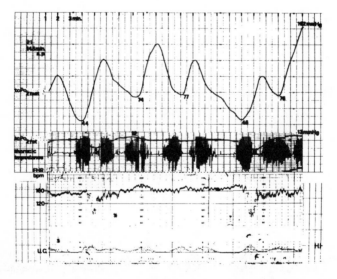

FIGURE 18a. Continuous recording of maternal transcutaneous oxygen tension ($tcPO_2$mat), fetal oxygen tension ($tcPO_2$fet), thoracic impedance, fetal heart rate (FHR), and uterine contractions (UC) in a primipara 120 minutes before spontaneous delivery of an infant with an Apgar 7. The same pattern was seen for 90 minutes during which there were 22 contractions that provoked marked hyperventilation followed by hypoventilation or apnea between contractions. With the parturient breathing air, during and after the 1st and 4th periods of hyperventilation the $tcPO_2$mat fell to 44 and 46, with a consequent fall in $tcPO_2$fet and variable decelerations. The record illustrates the value of supplementary oxygen given during other periods in preventing the $tcPO_2$mat from falling below 70 mm Hg, which was found to be the critical level below which deleterious fetal effects were noted. (Courtesy of Huch, A., et al.: Br. J. Obstet. Gynaecol. 84S1:1, 1977.)

It has been shown that partial pain relief achieved with narcotics reduces the degree of maternal hyperventilation during the contraction so that $PaCO_2$ remains about 25 mm Hg, but during uterine relaxation, the mild relative hypo-

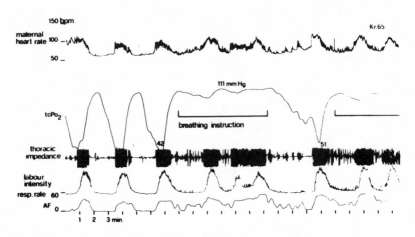

FIGURE 18b. Continuous recording of maternal heart rate, $tcPO_2$, thoracic impedance, uterine pressure, and respiratory rate after the parturient has been given 100 mg meperidine intramuscularly. With each uterine contraction there was marked hyperventilation that caused $tcPO_2$ to increase to 110 mm Hg, but then fall to very low levels as a result of the marked respiratory alkalosis and the respiratory depressant effect of the meperidine. The large falls in PO_2 were avoided by giving the parturient breathing instructions during the relaxation period. (Courtesy of Peabody, J.L.: Clinics in Pharmacology 6:109, 1979.)

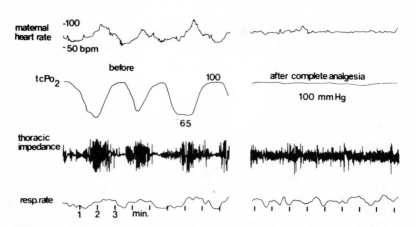

FIGURE 19. Polygraph recording of maternal heart rate, transcutaneous oxygen tension, thoracic impedance, and respiratory rate during labor. Before the induction of epidural analgesia, the pain of uterine contractions caused marked hyperventilation and consequent increase in $tcPO_2$mat to 100, which fell to 65–70 mm Hg between contractions. After complete epidural analgesia, all curves were more regular, and $tcPO_2$ was maintained at a stable 100 mg Hg. (Courtesy of Peabody, J.L.; Clinics in Pharmacology 6:109, 1979).

capnea and the depressant effects of the narcotic will result in hypoxemia which can be prevented by giving the patient breathing instructions during the relaxation period (Figure 18b). In contrast, complete pain relief achieved with extradural analgesia prevents the transient period of hyperventilation during contractions and hypoventilation during relaxation, and $PaCO_2$ remains about 30–32 mm Hg and PaO_2 about 100 mm Hg (Figure 19).

Clinical Implications

The anatomic changes are conducive to respiratory obstruction of the nasal passage, to an increased hazard of intubation, and to misinterpretation of physical findings. Special care must be taken in applying a face mask so that the patient is permitted to breathe through the mouth: nasopharyngeal tubes must be well lubricated and inserted carefully to avoid abrasion of the mucous membrane, and laryngoscopy and tracheal intubation must be performed skillfully and atraumatically.

Changes in lung volumes and ventilation increase the efficiency of gaseous transfer between maternal blood and alveolar air so that tension of CO_2 is decreased and that of oxygen is increased. These, in turn, enhance the transfer of these gases between the mother and the fetus. On the other hand, these changes make gravidas more susceptible to more rapid changes in respiratory blood gas levels during respiratory complications than are nonpregnant patients. Hypoventilation, breath-holding, or respiratory obstruction will produce hypoxia, hypercarbia, and respiratory acidosis more readily in the gravida than in the nonpregnant woman. For example, even skillful tracheal intubation in a parturient breathing air, frequently causes arterial oxygen tension to fall to 50–60 mm Hg after only 30 seconds of apnea. The tendency for rapid development of hypoxia is enhanced by high oxygen consumption during labor. Conversely, moderate to severe hyperventilation achieved spontaneously by the awake parturient or produced by an anesthetist through excessive positive pressure ventilation during general anesthesia can quickly lead to severe respiratory alkalosis which is often associated with decrease in cerebral blood flow and uterine blood flow and shift of the maternal oxygen dissociation curve to the left. Significant decrease in cerebral blood flow may produce a transient mental effect and analgesia and often is manifested by carpopedal spasm and other signs of tetany. The shift of the maternal oxygen dissociation curve and the decrease in uterine blood flow produce fetal hypoxia and metabolic acidosis.

The respiratory changes during pregnancy and labor also markedly influence the induction of, and recovery from, inhalation anesthesia. The increased alveolar ventilation speeds up the increase in alveolar concentration at the beginning of anesthesia and the decrease at the end, so that induction of, and emergence from, inhalation anesthesia is more rapid. This effect is less important with the less soluble gases such as nitrous oxide and cyclopropane than it is with the more soluble vapors such as diethyl ether, halothane, and enflurane.

Acid-base Balance

Total base decreases from the normal nonpregnant level of about 155 mEq/liter to about 148 mEq/liter to about 138 mEq/liter with a corresponding decrease in potassium, calcium, and magnesium. The total anions diminish commensurately, with the plasma bicarbonate decreasing from an average of 25 mEq/liter to 21 mEq/liter. *The plasma buffer base* (BB) which refers to the total available buffer and includes the bicarbonate, the protein, and the hemoglobin, decreases from a normal adult value of 47 mEq/liter to 42 mEq/liter and base excess decreases to -3.0 mEq/liter. In normal patients, the pH remains unchanged at 7.40, thus suggesting that in normal pregnancy there is a compensated alkali deficit, but in some gravidas there is a mild metabolic acidosis (pH 7.43).

OTHER PHYSIOLOGIC CHANGES

Gastrointestinal Function

In pregnancy, the stomach and intestines are progressively displaced cephalad by an enlarged uterus, and the axis of the stomach is shifted from a vertical to a horizontal with the pylorus displaced upward and posteriorly, thus slowing the emptying of gastric contents. There is usually slight diminution of gastric and intestinal tone and motility, a relative mild hypochlorhydria, and occasional development of reverse currents that carry material cephalad into the esophagous. Toward term there is an increased intragastric pressure, particularly in lithotomy and Trendelenburg positions, but this is usually exceeded by the increase in the opening pressure of the gastroesophageal sphincter so that in most unmedicated gravidas the risk of regurgitation is not enhanced. On the other hand, the incidence of hiatal hernia is increased during pregnancy, especially in elderly women, and this is associated with the regurgitation of acid stomach contents with consequent heartburn, esophagitis, and dysphagia.

During labor, the pain of uterine conractions and any associated anxiety and stress produce segmental and suprasegmental reflex inhibition of gastrointestinal motility and function with consequent significant delay in gastric emptying. These reflex effects of nociception are aggravated in the recumbent position and by most of the systemic analgesics and related drugs used for obstetric pain relief. This combined effect of pain and depressant drugs may cause food and even fluid other than water to be retained for as long as 36 hours during which swallowed air and gastric juices accumulate progressively with the pH of stomach contents decreasing below the critical value of 2.5 in most gravidas. The administration of general anesthesia and of muscle relaxants carries the serious risk of regurgitation and aspiration of gastric contents in all gravidas by obtunding the protective reflexes, increasing intra-abdominal pressure (succynlcholine-induced fasiculations) and relaxing the cricopharyngeal sphincter. Therefore, it is mandatory that parturients, particularly those who may require a general anesthetic, be give oral antacids (15 ml of magnesium tricilicate) every 3 hours during labor for those who are to deliver vaginally and 2 doses before cesarean section, with the first given 30 minutes and the second 10 minutes before induction of anesthesia.

Renal Function

During pregnancy, there is a gradual dilation of the renal pelves and calyces and ureters with a decrease in muscular tone and rhythmicity, resulting in an increase in urinary tract dead space. There is also a progressive increase in glomerular filtration rate (GFR) affecting renal plasma flow (RPF), filtration fraction, and tubular reabsorption. The rate of urine formation is increased because of the augemented load of excretory products. The increased GFR and RPF cause the urea nitrogen (BUN) to decrease from the nonpregnant level of 8–9 mg % to 5 mg % and creatinine from 0.46 mg % to 0.30 mg %. Therefore, if the gravida at term has a BUN or creatinine in the nonpregnant range, impairment of renal function should be suspected, and potentially nephrotoxic anesthetics such as methoxyflurane should be avoided. During the last trimester of pregnancy, the progressive compression of the lower aorta and its branches in the supine position causes a reduction of 20% in RPF and GFR and 60% in urine volume and excretion of sodium and chloride.

Hepatic Function

Several of the liver function tests are deranged during normal pregnancy, but the liver performs its function without difficulty. Hepatic blood flow is normal, but blood flow in relation to total blood volume is decreased. Moreover, the ability of the liver to eliminate bromsulphalein is more readily impaired by anesthetic agents in the gravida than in the nonpregnant state.

Endocrine System

Endocrine changes, other than persistence of corpus luteum and placental production of estrogen, progesterone, and chorionic gonadotropin include the following: (a) hyperplasia of the thyroid and parathyroid glands; (b) marked hypertrophy to double its size of the anterior lobe of the pituitary gland and increase in activity without increase in size of the posterior lobe; (c) enlargement of the adrenal glands and marked increase in the activity of the adrenal cortex manifested by increased plasma levels of 17-hydroxycorticosteroids, a threefold increase in aldosterone secretion and excretion, combined with a decrease in the circulating eosinophiles. The urinary excretion of neutral 17-ketosteroids remains within normal range.

Metabolism

During pregnancy, there is a progressive increase in basal metabolic rate and oxygen consumption (which at term is 20% above normal), retention and storage of water, protein, and minerals, retention of salts and the acquisition of fat. During parturition, there is a further significant increase in metabolism and oxygen consumption to meet the increased work by the uterus, and during the second stage, the additional work consequent to the bearing down efforts. Parturients who have inadequate pain relief have greater oxygen consumption than those who have complete pain relief, and most of the former will develop a progressive metabolic acidosis and a steady rise in the level of concentration of free fatty acids and other endocrine responses to pain (Chapter 3).

PSYCHOLOGIC EFFECTS OF PREGNANCY AND ANESTHESIA

During pregnancy and labor, the patient may be disturbed by apprehension, anxiety, fear, and other affective reactions that not only modify her emotional well-being, but also may further increase heart rate, cardiac output and blood pressure, and may even produce other psychosomatic effects. She may be disturbed by fear of the unknown, of death, of suffering, of mutilation, of possible complications, or concern for her own condition or that of her fetus. Unless properly prepared, the impending anesthetic may provoke anxiety and fear of possible anesthetic complications or death, or the fear that the anesthesia will cause loss of senses and inhibitions that might cause the patient to perform irresponsible acts or betray secrets. Dreams during anesthesia may evoke an immediate abnormal physical reaction or may produce deleterious psychologic effects following anesthetization. Since dreams are responses to internal or external stimuli that disturb sleep, they are frequently provoked by premature preparation and operation by the obstetrician and by loud noises or comments made during the induction of, and emergence from, general anesthesia.

CHAPTER 2. PHYSIOLOGY AND PHARMACOLOGY OF THE PLACENTA, FETUS AND NEWBORN

The placenta plays a vital role in the growth and development of the fetus and in maintaining homeostasis by functioning as the fetal lung, kidney, liver, and intestines. It is also a potent endocrine organ responsible for many of the maternal changes that occur during pregnancy, and it critically influences uterine contractility. The efficiency of the placenta in maintaining fetal homeostasis and in determining the fetal and neonatal effects of anesthetics and related drugs given to the mother is dependent upon: (1) uteroplacental circulation; (2) placental transfer; and (3) fetal circulation and the fetal distribution, tissue uptake, and excretion of drugs. These three aspects and the physiology of the newborn will be briefly summarized in this chapter.

THE PLACENTA

Uteroplacental Circulation

The uteroplacental circulation is responsible for bringing nutritive materials and oxygen to the fetus and taking away carbon dioxide and other fetal waste products. Uterine blood flow in the human gravida at term is about 700 ml/min representing 10% of the cardiac output. Of this, 70–85% (500–625 ml) passes through the intervillous space, and the remainder supplies the myometrium. The umbilical blood flow at term, before labor, is said to be about 500–600 ml–min, representing about 50% of the combined ventricular output. About 400–500 ml participate in the exchange with the maternal blood while the remainder does not, either because it passes through vascular shunts within the fetal side of the placenta or it does not approach closely enough to maternal blood to exchange with it. At delivery, the acute events apparently decrease umbilical blood flow to about 250–300 ml–min.

The dynamics of the maternal side of the circulation are such as to produce a *vis a tergo* effect that favors unimpeded flow from maternal uterine arteries where the mean arterial pressure is about 80 mm Hg to the spiral arteries which end as open vessels in the intervillous space. The blood enters the intervillous space in fountain-like "spurts" at a pressure of 70–80 mm Hg which is considerably higher than the 10 mm Hg pressure prevailing in the intervillous space. The maternal blood bathes fetal villi and their capillaries and is drained by venous channels which have still lower pressures (5 mm Hg).

The uterine circulation is under a strong alpha adrenergic receptor control and a mild beta control so that pain and stress and the consequent liberation of norepinephrine increase uterine vascular resistance and decrease blood flow. Moreover, the uterine circulation acts as a critically damped system without any degree of autoregulation. Therefore, with the exception of stimulation acting through these receptors, the uterine blood flow depends on the perfusing pressure with a critical closing pressure of about 30 mm Hg. Consequently, a decrease in the driving (perfusing) pressure decreases uterine blood flow and the number and size of "spurts." A decrease in the driving pressure resulting from either a rise in intervillous pressure or a fall in end-spiral artery pressure results from maternal hypotension or aortoiliac compression by the uterus or both.

Aortoiliac compression is greatly exaggerated in the presence of maternal hypotension, often resulting in marked decrease of intervillous perfusion. Maternal hypotension produced by sympathetic blockade of regional anesthesia or cardiovascular depression by general anesthesia, supine hypotension, and/or hemorrhage is probably the most frequent cause of decreased perfusion and consequent fetal distress. A rise in intervillous pressure is usually due to uterine contractions but may also be caused by hypertonus consequent to tetanic contraction, over-stimulation with oxytocin, or a ruptured placenta. Endogenous catecholamine release produced by pain and stress and/or the exogenous administration of vasoconstrictors with predominant alpha adrenergic action also markedly decrease uterine blood flow.

Uterine contractions can decrease perfusion by increasing intra-amniotic pressure or exaggerating the aorto-iliac compression or both. Uterine contractions of 20 mm Hg or less have little or no effect on intervillous perfusion, contractions of 20 to 30 mm Hg decrease it by as much as 50%, while contractions greater than 50 mm Hg produce complete cessation of intervillous perfusion. The frequently recurring contractions of active labor and the consequent recurring, albeit brief, impairment of intervillous perfusion and blood gas transfer, result in mild degrees of fetal respiratory acidosis and hypoxemia. Consequently, normal birth is an asphyxial process that, under normal circumstances, is sufficiently mild to be beneficial because the slight hypercapnia and hypoxia help the newborn to establish and maintain regular breathing. However, this birth asphyxia is markedly aggravated by an abnormal increase in uterine contractility, maternal hypotension, compression of the umbilical cord, or other pathologic processes of the placenta that chronically decrease uterine and umbilical blood flows and thus markedly interfere with placental transfer. In such circumstances, the severe birth asphyxia causes neonatal depression and impairs the newborn's ability for extrauterine adaption. The neonatal depressant effects of severe birth asphyxia are potentiated by sedative, narcotics, and other depressant drugs given to the mother for pain relief.

Vasopressors used to treat maternal hypotension may impair uterine blood flow. This is particularly true of those drugs that have an alpha adrenergic stimulating action (e.g., methoxamine, phenylephrine), all of which have been shown to decrease uterine blood flow and intervillous perfusion as reflected by a decrease in fetal PaO_2 and pH and an increase in $PaCO_2$. (See Figure 38, p. 92.)

As mentioned in the preceding chapter, maternal hyperventilation, either voluntary by the parturient or induced by controlled respiration during general anesthesia, produces a respiratory alkalosis and a consequent decrease in uterine blood flow. Moreover, severe maternal hypoxia produces a marked increase in uterine vascular resistance with a consequent severe decrease in uterine blood flow.

Placental Transfer

In the human at term, the placental membrane consists of 3 unicellular layers about 3.5μ thick and a total surface area of about 11 M^2. Placental transfer is achieved by: (a) simple diffusion; (b) facilitated diffusion; (c) active transport, which includes active enzymatic transfer and enzymatic destruction; and (d) through special processes, including pinocytosis and breaks in the placenta villi. Oxygen, carbon dioxide, and other catabolic products, as well as sedatives, narcotics, and general and local anesthetics, are transferred by simple diffusion, although there is some recent evidence that oxygen may be transferred by a process of facilitated diffusion. Factors that influence the transfer of oxygen and carbon dioxide include the concentration gradient, dissociation curves, and the capacity of maternal-fetal blood for these gases, as well as the functional capacity and thickness of the membrane which in certain pathologic states are decreased and increased, respectively, and maternal and fetal blood flow on both sides of

TABLE 3. FACTORS INFLUENCING TRANSFER OF DRUGS ACROSS THE PLACENTA

DRUG FACTORS	MATERNAL FACTORS	FETAL FACTORS
1. Degree of ionization	1. Maternal blood volume	1. Fetal liver
2. Lipid solubility	2. Elimination of drug from maternal circulation	2. Progressive dilution of blood en route to fetal brain
3. Binding to plasma proteins and red cells	3. Nonhomogenicity of blood in intervillous space	3. Extensive shunting in fetal circulation
4. Concentration gradient across the membrane	4. Separation of maternal from fetal circulation	4. Immaturity of the brain
5. Molecular weight	5. Uteroplacental blood flow	5. Immature enzymatic systems
6. Method of administration	6. Uterine contractions	6. Fetal plasma, red cells, and pH
7. Drug interaction		7. Compression of umbilical cord during delivery
8. Drug metabolites		
9. Tissue binding		

the placenta. (See Figures 20, 21, and Table 3). Nutrients such as glucone, glucose, amino acids, and vitamins move by active transport; hormones and other substances that maintain pregnancy and fetal growth cross by slow diffusion; and red cells, proteins, and other substances of immunologic import leak through pores in the placenta.

The rate of diffusion of drugs is governed by physicochemical factors including degree of ionization and lipid solubility of the drug, protein binding, the concentration gradient (difference in concentration of the drug on both sides of the membrance), and molecular weight, as well as the area and thickness of the membrane and fetal and maternal blood flow. Nonionized drugs with high lipid solubility are transferred rapidly, whereas lipid insoluble drugs penetrate poorly, despite a low degree of ionization. Most drugs used in anesthesia are transferred rapidly across the placental membrane and can achieve equilibrium between maternal and fetal blood in a matter of minutes, depending on the dose given to the mother.

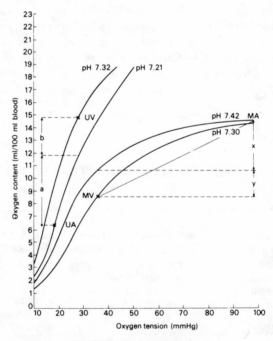

FIGURE 20. Portrayal of the major determinants of oxygen transfer from mother to fetus. The curves relate to the association between oxygen tension and oxygen content for maternal artery (MA) and maternal vein (MV) blood at pH values 7.42 and 7.30, respectively, and to umbilical vein (UV) and umbilical artery (UA) blood at pH values 7.32 and 7.21, respectively; with x, the volume of oxygen donated by maternal blood in response to the pressure gradient; y, the volume of oxygen donated by maternal blood as a result of the Bohr effect; a, the volume of oxygen received by fetal blood as a result of the pressure gradient; and b, the volume of oxyen received by fetal blood as a result of the Bohr effect. (Courtesy of Crawford, J.S.: *Obstetric Anaesthesia*, Oxford, Blackwell Scientific Publications, 1978.)

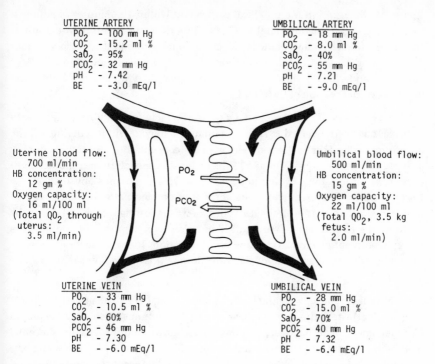

UTERINE ARTERY
```
PO2   - 100 mm Hg
CO2   - 15.2 ml %
SaO2  - 95%
PCO2  - 32 mm Hg
pH    - 7.42
BE    - -3.0 mEq/1
```

UMBILICAL ARTERY
```
PO2   - 18 mm Hg
CO2   - 8.0 ml %
SaO2  - 40%
PCO2  - 55 mm Hg
pH    - 7.21
BE    - -9.0 mEq/1
```

Uterine blood flow:
    700 ml/min
HB concentration:
    12 gm %
Oxygen capacity:
    16 ml/100 ml
(Total QO2 through
  uterus:
    3.5 ml/min)

PO2

PCO2

Umbilical blood flow:
    500 ml/min
HB concentration:
    15 gm %
Oxygen capacity:
    22 ml/100 ml
(Total QO2, 3.5 kg
  fetus:
    2.0 ml/min)

UTERINE VEIN
```
PO2   - 33 mm Hg
CO2   - 10.5 ml %
SaO2  - 60%
PCO2  - 46 mm Hg
pH    - 7.30
BE    - -6.0 mEq/1
```

UMBILICAL VEIN
```
PO2   - 28 mm Hg
CO2   - 15.0 ml %
SaO2  - 70%
PCO2  - 40 mm Hg
pH    - 7.32
BE    - -6.4 mEq/1
```

FIGURE 21. The placental transfer of oxygen and carbon dioxide between maternal and fetal-placental blood. The values were derived from various reports based on animal and human studies at term gestation. It is likely that the oxygenation and acid-base status of the undisturbed (unstudied) fetus are better than indicated by the figures in this illustration. (Modified from and courtesy of Bonica, J.J.: *Principles and Practice of Obstetric Analgesia and Anesthesia,* Philadelphia, F.A. Davis Company, 1967.)

Inhalation Agents. Inhalation anesthetics pass through the placental membrane rapidly. Their high speed of transfer is related to their rapid rates of diffusion, relatively high fat solubility, and usually low molecular weight. Administered in analgesic concentration with the mother awake, oriented, and cooperative, no significant depression of the newborn is seen, regardless of the duration of administration. However, when inhalation agents are administered in anesthetic concentrations, the degree of neonatal depression is proportionate to the depth and duration of maternal anesthesia.

Nitrous oxide is rapidly transferred so that in less than 4 minutes the fetal/maternal nitrous oxide-oxygen concentration reaches the highest level of 80%. Lower fetal/maternal ratios are related to placental or cord complications. Uptake of the agent by fetal tissues is also rapid with umbilical artery-vein blood nitrous oxide concentration ratio increasing progressively with duration of anesthesia and achieving an 87% equilibration within 14–19 minutes.

Cyclopropane, diethyl ether, trichloroethylene, and other older inhalation agents can be found in the umbilical cord blood within 1½ minutes of administration. Both maternal and fetal levels of these drugs rise with the duration of anesthesia. Similarly, **halothane** is detectable in fetal umbilical vein blood within 2 minutes of the start of administration. By using low concentrations (0.5% of halothane and 25–50% nitrous oxide for cesarean section), there is little or no time-related depression of the infant.

Methoxyflurane (Penthrane), an agent used widely for obstetric analgesia-anesthesia, has been detected in newborn infants delivered within 2 minutes of the beginning of the administration. The average concentration of methoxyflurane in umbilical vein blood is about 50% of maternal concentration in patients anesthetized for less than 10 minutes and about 75% in patients anesthetized for 10–15 minutes. The methoxyflurane content of umbilical artery blood is significantly lower than that of umbilical vein blood, suggesting a high uptake of the agent by the fetal tissues. Free fluoride has also been demonstrated in mothers and newborns after methoxyflurane administration. It would seem prudent to minimize the total amount of methoxyflurane that is administered to the mother.

Barbiturates. The slow-acting barbiturates, barbital (Veronal) and phenobarbital (Luminal), and the intermediate acting barbiturates such as amobarbital (Amytal) and vinbarbital (Delvinal) have been shown to transverse the placental membrane rapidly and achieve equilibrium in 5–20 minutes. The fast-acting barbiturates, pentobarbital (Nembutal) and secobarbital (Seconal), can be detected in fetal blood within 1 minute of intravenous administration to the mother, and equilibrium is established between mother and infant within 3–5 minutes.

The initial studies of the placental transfer of thiopental sodium (Pentothal) suggested that only minute amounts of the drug were found in the newborn infant during the first 5–7 minutes, and equilibrium between maternal and fetal blood was reached only after 10–12 minutes. On the basis of these data, the misconception developed among clinicians that thiopental could be given without affecting the baby if delivery was achieved within 8 minutes. However, subsequent studies showed that the drug passes the membrane within seconds, achieves the highest concentration in umbilical vein blood within 1½–2 minutes of the injection, and then falls exponentially (Figure 22).

Currently, barbiturates are rarely used for sedation during labor, but thiopental and ultra-short acting barbiturates given intravenously are used for the induction of balanced general anesthesia. Although older studies failed to show correlation between the concentration of the drug in the umbilical vein and neonatal depression or the depth of maternal anesthesia, more recent studies in which neurobehavioral assessment was used have revealed a depressant effect that lasts for about 48 hours. If thiopental is given in doses of 4 mg/kg or greater, significant neonatal depression occurs. However, with doses of 3 mg/kg or less given as a single induction dose, no neonatal depression occurs. Following intravenous administration of thiopental, the concentration is low in fetal brain and

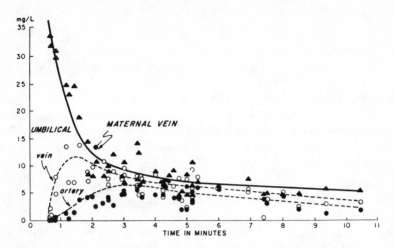

FIGURE 22. The level of thiopental in maternal vein, umbilical vein, and umbilical artery following injection of a single dose of 4 mg/kg for induction of anesthesia. Note the rapid decay of the maternal venous blood level and the rapid transfer to the fetus. (Courtesy of Kosaka, Y., et al.: Anesthesiology 31:489, 1969).

spinal cord but high in liver and subcutaneous fat, thus demonstrating the efficacy of the liver and the dilution factor in decreasing the concentration of a drug that reaches the brain.

The amount of thiopental or any other systemic drug transferred to the fetus can be decreased by injecting the drug IV at the beginning of the uterine contraction. By the time the bolus of the drug goes through the maternal central circulation into the uterine arteries, the uterine contraction would be at its peak and, consequently, intervillous perfusion is either imparied or totally arrested so that lesser amounts or no drug is transferred during this first circulation time. By the time of the second and subsequent circulations, the maternal level of the thiopental is much lower, resulting in lesser amounts of placental transfer.

Tranquilizers. Chloropromazine (Thorazine), promethazine (Phenergan), and promazine (Sparine) can be found in the umbilical vein blood within 1½–2 minutes of intravenous administration to the mother with a maximum fetal concentration occurring during the ensuing 2–3 minutes. Most studies have shown that the concentration in fetal blood is always lower than that in maternal blood. Moreover, a significantly greater proportion of these drugs given to the mother is passed to the fetus after intravenous than after intramuscular administration.

The benzodiazepines initially were considered to be without untoward effects, but later studies showed that *diazepam* produces neonatal hypothermia and hypotonia. Moreover, the placental transfer and fetal protein binding of diazepam are so extensive that its level is higher in fetal blood and fetal tissues than those of the mother. Although other members of this group of drugs are also transferred in significant amounts, they do not share the neonatal effects of diazepam.

Ketamine. Ketamine, which can be used for tranquilization-analgesia during labor and vaginal delivery or as an intravenous induction agent for cesarean section, is transferred rapidly across the placenta, and within a few minutes after intraveous injection there is equilibration between maternal and fetal blood. Used in large doses (2 mg/kg), it causes neonatal depression of nonasphyxial origin and may cause maternal hypertension and uterine hypertonicity, but, when used in doses of 0.5 mg/kg, these untoward effects are not seen.

Narcotics. Meperidine reaches the umbilical vein blood within 30 seconds of intravenous administration to the mother in levels approaching 70% of maternal values. This ratio of umbilical venous to maternal arterial concentration is maintained for about 5–10 minutes, and following this there is a rapid decay. Meperidine concentrations are higher in the umbilical vein than in the umbilical artery for the first 3–5 minutes, but thereafter the levels become virtually the same. The maternal metabolites of meperidine also cross the placenta. Although most studies have shown no correlation between the Apgar scores and the clinical condition of the infant and the level of meperidine in neonatal plasma, neurobehavioral assessment reveals neonatal depression for 4–8 hours. Pentazocine, the narcotic with weak opiate antagonist properties, has been found in cord blood in levels that are 40–70% of maternal levels. Other narcotics undoubtedly behave similarly. Naloxone (Narcan) also passes the placental membrane rapidly; this is not unexpected, since this and other antagonists represent only slight modification in the molecular structure of narcotics.

Skeletal Muscle Relaxants. At normal pH range, muscle relaxants are highly ionized and posses a low degree of lipid solubility. Because of these properties, these agents pass through the placental membrane with great difficulty. Usual clinical doses have no demonstrable effects on the newborn, and, with the exception of gallamine, significant quantities of the drugs cannot be detected in the infant's blood stream. If massive doses of these drugs (5–10 times or more of therapeutic doses) are injected, resulting in an extremely high concentration gradient across the placenta, the relaxants may be found in cord blood and may produce clinical effects in the newborn.

Local Anesthetics. Local anesthetics pass through the placental membrane and reach the infant quickly. They are found in maternal and fetal blood within 3–5 minutes of injection, reach peak levels 15–30 minutes thereafter, and then there is a rapid decay as uptake by a vessel-rich group occurs. The ratio of fetal-maternal blood levels is about one with Prilocaine (Citanest), 0.6–0.8 with lidocaine (Xylocaine) and mepivacaine (Carbocaine), 0.3–0.5 with bupivacaine (Marcaine), and 0.2–0.4 with etidocaine (Duranest). This difference is due to the degree of protein binding capacity of each local anesthetic, with bupivacaine and etidocaine having the highest capacity, prilocaine the lowest, and the values of lidocane and mepivacaine being intermediate. (See Table 9, p. 87.)

In constrast to other local anesthetics, no significant levels of 2-chloroprocaine (Nesacaine) can be detected in fetal blood because this drug is rapidly hydrolized by plasma pseudocholinesterase to 2-chloro-p-aminobenzoic acid and diethyl-aminoethanol, and only these nontoxic breakdown products reach the fetal circulation. The *in vitro* half-life of 2-chloroprocaine is 22 sec in maternal blood and 44 sec in fetal blood.

Fetal electrocardiography and fetal heart rate (FHR) measurements show that there is an initial stabilization of the beat-to-beat interval of FHR that is a sign of the loss of integrity of the fetal autonomic nervous system. The fetal toxic effects from excessive doses of local anesthetics are depression of the nervous system and myocardium and consequent arterial hypotension. Fetal bradycardia is seen generally only with very high doses of local anesthetics administered to the fetus directly or in association with paracervical block. The decrease in fetal heart rate beat-to-beat variability following maternal epidural analgesia is transient and unassociated with fetal or neonatal depression. Neurobehavioral assessment studies have shown that, when used in analgesic concentrations, bupivacaine and chloroprocaine have no depressant effect compared to a control group of infants whose mothers received no anesthesia or subarachnoid block. In contrast, the use of 1.5% mepivacaine or lidocaine produced muscular hypotonia, diminished motor reflex, decreased rooting activity, and sporadic alteration response to repetitive stimulation during the first 8 hours of life, and these effects paralleled the peak levels of the local anesthetic in the infant's blood. Since epidural analgesia can be achieved with 0.5–1.0%, it is likely that much less depression of the newborn results with these optimal concentrations.

FETAL PHYSIOLOGY AND PHARMACOLOGY

The response of the fetus and newborn to drugs administered to the mother is related mainly to the concentration achieved and maintained in its central nervous system and, to a lesser extent, in the myocardium, the two vital organs that are the special targets of depressant action. This is, in turn, influenced by the fetal circulation and, consequently, the fetal distribution, tissue uptake, drug metabolism, and excretion. The blood from the placenta with an 80% oxygen saturation is conveyed to the fetus via the umbilical vein that divides below the liver into two branches, a smaller branch, which breaks up into several branches that empty into the liver, and the larger ductus venosus, which bypasses the liver and drains into the inferior vena cava (Figure 23a). Under normal conditions, 50–60% of the umbilical vein blood drains through the ductus venosus, but, in the presence of moderately severe acidosis and hypoxemia, this increases to as much as 80–90%. The higher oxygenated blood from the ductus venosus and liver that empties into the inferior vena cava mixes with desaturated (25%) blood coming from the lower part of the body so that the blood in the inferior vena cava above the liver is about 65–70% saturated. Most of this blood bypasses the right auricle and passes through the foramen ovale to the left ventricle which then pumps it to the aorta, with most of the still highly oxygenated blood (60–65%) passing to the coronary and cerebral circulation. The desaturated blood (30%) from the upper part of the body drains into the superior vena cava which diverts it directly to the right ventricle that pumps it to the pulmonary artery, with 70% of the blood bypassing the lung via the ductus arteriosus to the aorta for reoxygenation by the placenta. These three shunts—ductus venosus, foramen ovale, and ductus arteriosus—are crucial to the well-being of the fetus, and, in the presence of diminishing placental supply of oxygen, the umbilical blood flow to the heart and brain will be increased by diversion of blood from the liver, by the enlarging ductus venosus, and by diversion of blood from the pulmonary circulation (which responds by marked vasoconstriction in the presence of asphyxia and release of catecholamines) through the foramen ovale and ductus arteriosus.

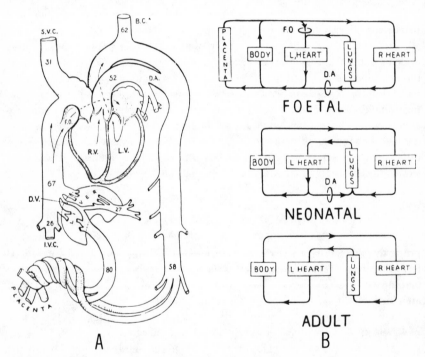

FIGURE 23. Fetal circulation (left) and changes at birth (right). In the fetal circulation, the saturation is highest in the inferior vena cava (IVC) above the liver and progressively decreases in the brachiocephalic artery (BCA) and aorta, and is lowest in the inferior vena cava below the liver. RV, right ventricle; DV, ductus venosus; DA, ductus arteriosus; SVC, superior vena cava; LV, left ventricle; FO, foramen ovale. The *diagram on the right* shows the circulation of the fetus (upper diagram) in which both ventricles work in parallel to drive blood from the great veins to the arteries. Transitional circulation (middle) is present during the first day or two of life, when the foramen ovale is closed but the ductus arteriosus is still open. Adult circulation (lower) which results after the ductus arteriosus closes; the blood is pumped through the lungs and body by the two ventricles operating in series. (Courtesy of Born, G., et al.: Sympos. Quant. Biol. 19:102, 1954.)

Because of this peculiar fetal circulation, once the drug passes through the placental membrane and reaches the umbilical circulation, concentration gradients are developed as this blood mixes with the blood coming from other parts of the fetal body.

The rate of entry of drugs into the brain is primarily governed by the degree of lipoid solubility of the nonionized drug molecules because the blood-brain barrier is like a lipoid membrane. In the fetus and newborn, there is an increase in the permeability of the blood-brain barrier to drugs. The rate of transfer across the blood-brain barrier is also related to the extent of protein binding that occurs between a given substance and plasma proteins. Finally, hypercapnia and hypoxia markedly increase cerebral permeability to many drugs: hypocapnia reduces it, but hyperoxia has no effect.

Fetal Drug Metabolism and Excretion

Disposition of drugs by the fetus is less efficient than in the adult as many of the enzyme systems essential for the metbolism of drugs are immature and some are absent. Nevertheless, human fetal liver samples have very high levels of cytochrome P-450, a major drug metabolizing enzyme, which are present as early as the 14th week of gestation. Whether significant *in utero* fetal hepatic metabolism of drug occurs is uncertain, but there is some evidence that phenobarbital can induce glucuronyl transferase activity in the fetal liver following its administration to the mother, as suggested by the fact that newborns of mothers given this drug show a marked decrease in bilirubin level. These include enzymes which metabolize bartiburates used for sedation or induction of general anesthesia, local anesthetics, some narcotics, and a variety of other drugs. Since renal function is less efficient in the fetus than in the adult, it is likely that those drugs primarily excreted by the kidney, such as barbital, may have a long residual effect in the fetus. As a result of these factors, the depressant effects of narcotics, barbiturates, and promethazine persist for many hours and as long as 2–4 days after birth.

PHYSIOLOGY OF THE NEWBORN

Respiration

The onset and maintenance of adequate ventilation of the newborn require: (1) ample respiratory stimuli; (2) an undepressed respiratory center; (3) normal lung structure, including alveoli that are able to receive air and distend appropriately, a pulmonary capillary bed sufficiently mature to receive and absorb oxygen, and a normal diffusing membrane; (4) a normal thoracic cage and respiratory neuromuscular mechanism; (5) a clear, unobstructed airway; (6) an ample supply of oxygen; and (7) a cardiovascular system that functions adequately. Immediately after birth the surface tension in the respiratory tract must be overcome and the blood circulation must change from the fetal to the transitional form. Most infants have these requirements and breathe spontaneously within seconds of delivery. Although the fetus breathes *in utero*, at birth the newborn has to establish regular sustained respiration which results from stimulation of the respiratory center by intensive nonrespiratory neuronal stimulation provoked by exposure to extrauterine existence and the increasing carbon dioxide and mild acidosis of birth asphyxia.

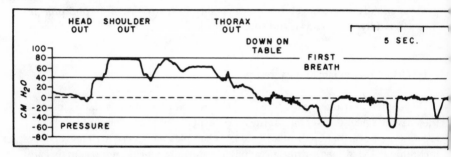

FIGURE 24a. Intrathoracic pressure changes produced during and after delivery as measured by the intraesophageal catheter technique. Note the marked increase in intrathoracic pressure during the time the thorax is passing through birth canal and the significant negative pressure produced by the first and subsequent breaths. (Modified from the courtesy of Karlberg, P.: J. Pediat. 56:585, 1960.)

During birth, the fetal chest is significantly compressed as it passes through the birth canal by pressures varying from 35–95 cm H_2O. This results in diminution of the volume of the thoracic cavity. As soon as the head is delivered, the respiratory tract is exposed to lower atmospheric pressure, resulting in a significant pressure gradient that tends to promote drainage of the amniotic fluid from the air passages to the outside (Figure 24a). As soon as the trunk of the newborn is delivered, the compressed forces are released as the pressure drops almost to zero almost immediately, and the elasticity of the thorax causes recoil of the thoracic cavity. As the lungs reexpand, the amniotic fluid contained in the upper airway passage is drawn backward into the respiratory tract. Since some of the fluid was already expelled, air must be sucked in, at least into the upper part of the respiratory tract and the major bronchi. The volume inspired is about 20–40 ml and may even go as high as 70 ml. With the first inspiratory effort, the undepressed newborn frequently develops a negative intrathoracic pressure of about -45 cm H_2O (range -20 to -70 cm H_2O) causing 40 to 70 ml of air to be drawn in (Figure 24b). The first inspiration is usually followed by a cry as the infant expires against a partially closed glottis. This creates a positive intrathoracic pressure of up to 40 cm H_2O and prevents an egress of about half of the inspired air, the remainder being left to build up the residual volume. The first minute is characterized by single, irregular breaths followed by a period of transitional irregular breathing that lasts about 1–10 minutes. Following this period, normal infants develop a regular breathing pattern, and the respiratory rate increases to 40–50 breaths per minute. During the initial several breaths, pressure changes and tidal volumes are similar to those of the first breath, and the residual volume, functional residual capacity, and lung aeration increase progressively. Thereafter, a progressively smaller negative pressure is exerted, and smaller volumes are respired. At about the 5th to 10th minute after birth, respiration becomes quiet, and the mechanics of breathing are similar to those found later in the neonatal period when pressure changes are -2 cm H_2O during expiration and -7 cm H_2O during inspiration and tidal volume is 15 to 20 ml (Figure 25).

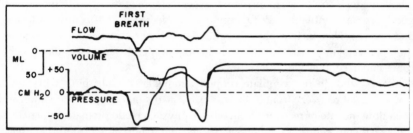

FIGURE 24b. The record of simultaneously recorded volume changes in intraesophageal pressure and airflow before, during, and after the first breath. Note the slight time lag between negative and intrathoracic pressure, airflow, and volume changes. (Modified from and courtesy of Karlberg, P.: J. Pediat. 56:585, 1960.)

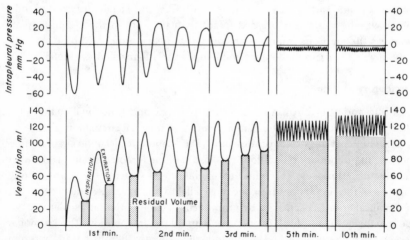

FIGURE 25. Ventilation during first minutes after birth. During first several breaths, pressure changes and tidal volumes are similar, and residual volume, functional residual capacity, and lung aeration increase progressively. Thereafter, a progressively smaller negative pressure is exerted, and smaller volumes are respired. After a few minutes, respiration becomes quiet, and the mechanics of breathing are similar to those found later in the neonatal period when pressure changes are -2 mm Hg during expiration and -7 mm Hg during inspiration, and tidal volume is 15–20 ml. (See text for details.) (Courtesy of Bonica, J.J.: *Principles and Practice of Obstetric Analgesia and Anesthesia* Philadelphia, F.A. Davis Company, 1967.)

The ventilation pattern of a vigorous newborn helps the infant to develop regular breathing and to recover from birth asphyxia that, as mentioned, occurs during all births. The rhythmic uterine contractions interfere with placental gas transfer so that all infants incur hypoxia and hypercarbia and mild acidosis. This is because of the rapid rate of oxygen desaturation of the blood and increase in CO_2 and fixed acids that accompany interference with respiratory gas exchange. The process is aggravated by cord compression, maternal hypotension, and other factors. The hypoxia that develops during birth inhibits the respiratory center but is offset by the sensory and metabolic stimulation. During the first few seconds after birth, the PCO_2 rises sharply, but, with the onset of transitional breathing, it falls rapidly and oxygen tension increases. However, the metabolic acidosis continues to increase for several more minutes. With the onset of good, regular ventilation, PCO_2 continues to decrease, PO_2 continues to rise, and recovery from birth asphyxia begins. The rate of recovery is at first rapid but then proceeds more slowly, and at 1–2 hours of life, the acid-base state has become stabilized. (See Figure 60a, p. 176.)

Infants who do not ventilate properly immediately after birth will have a slower rate of recovery from birth asphyxia. Factors that depress ventilation and thus slow the rate of recovery from birth asphyxia include prematurity, analgesics, anesthetics and other depressant drugs, and maternal or obstetric complications that impair uteroplacental blood flow and thus produce more serious birth asphyxia. Depressed infants are more acidotic and have higher serum potassium levels at birth than do vigorous infants. During the immediate postnatal period, a fall in pH and buffer base and the rise in PCO_2 and lactate are greater and of longer duration in the depressed infant than they are in the vigorous infant. Whereas the vigorous infant has recovered to near normal acid-base state by 1 hour of age, the depressed infant is still moderately to markedly acidotic.

Circulatory System

During and after birth, a series of morphologic and functional changes take place that drastically alter the hemodynamics of the fetal circulation (Figure 23b, p. 34). The most important of these are: (1) cessation of placental circulation; (2) increase in pulmonary blood flow; (3) closure of the foramen ovale; (4) closure of the ductus arteriosus; (5) transient alteration in systemic pressure; and (6) changes of the circulation from one in parallel to one in series. The rapid closure of umbilical arteries is effected by prompt contraction of their musculature. With the expansion of the lung incident to extrauterine respiration, the pulmonary vessels become uncoiled and dilate and consequently there is a profound diminution of vascular resistence and a four-fold increase in pulmonary blood flow. The increase in pulmonary venous return resulting from the augmented pulmonary circulation increases the pressure in the left atrium while, at the same time, there is a marked decrease in the pressure of the inferior vena cava resulting from reduced venous return consequent to obliteration of the umbilical vessels. This results in a sudden marked change in the pressure relationship between the left atrium and inferior vena cava which in turn causes functional closure of the foramen ovale within a minute or so of delivery, although it does not become sealed for several weeks. One hour after birth, the right-to-left shunt decreases, and for the next few hours there is a bidirectional shunt that subsequently becomes entirely left to right, and, by 15 hours of age, shunting of blood either becomes physiologically insignificant or ceases entirely. Functional closure of the ductus arteriosus is provoked by an increase in the oxygen tension in the blood flowing through it and occurs in 10–15 hours and is sealed in 3–4 weeks.

It is apparent that fetal circulation does not suddenly change into adult circulation in miniature immediately at birth. The transitional circulation is of great importance to survival during the first few hours or days of life when the newborn is striving to exist independently or when his lungs and heart have little reserve capacity. With functional closure of the foramen ovale and the ductus arteriosus, the two ventricles no longer work in parallel but rather in series, one to pump blood through the lungs and the other through the tissues. This results in a threefold increase in the output of each ventricle that, together with the marked increase in tone, greatly augments cardiac work and more than offsets the decrease caused by eliminating the placenta from the circulation.

The cardiac output of the newborn human infant ranges between 200 and 800 ml/min with an average of 500 ml/min or approximately 160 ml/kg/min. Following birth, the heart rate declines from an average of 140/min in the fetus at term to 110–115/min, with a minimum rate of 95/min and a maximum rate of 130/min. In the newborn, the systemic systolic pressure averages 70 mm Hg while the diastolic averages 45 mm Hg.

Thermoregulation

Thermoregulation in the newborn is accomplished by nonshivering thermogenesis and an increase in metabolic rate and oxygen consumption without muscular activity. Brown adipose tissue (so-called because of its rich vascular supply) which is responsible for this heat production is found in the interscapular area, axillae, perirenal area, and in the muscles and blood vessels of the neck and thoracic inlet. When the newborn is cold-stressed, large amounts of norepinephrine are released (in contrast to epinephrine in adults) and activate adipose tissue lipase which breaks down brown fat into triglycerides. The latter are then hydrolyzed to form glycerol and nonesterified fatty acids (NEFA). Then the NEFA are either oxidized to carbon dioxide, water, or are re-esterified to triglyceride. This oxidation is a highly exothermic reaction and is thought to be the resynthesis of triglycerides. Any interference with this mechanism would hinder the ability of the newborn to maintain his temperature through a cold-stress. Many drugs used for sedation and analgesia impair the newborn infant's ability to maintain temperature. These include reserpine, meperidine, and probably other narcotics, diazepam, large amounts of thiobarbiturates, and excessive amounts of local anesthetics.

CHAPTER 3. THE FORCES OF LABOR AND THE PAIN OF PARTURITION

The first part of this chapter contains a brief summary of the physiology of uterine contractions and the bearing-down efforts during labor and vaginal delivery and how these are affected by sedatives, systemic analgesics, and regional analgesia used for obstetric pain relief. The second part of the chapter summarizes the current concepts of the nature of pain of parturition.

PHYSIOLOGY OF THE FORCES OF LABOR

Delivery of the fetus is achieved by a delicate balance between the expulsive forces consisting of uterine contractions and the auxiliary forces (bearing down) on the one hand, and the resistance of the lower uterine segment, cervix, and perineum on the other. Since analgesia and anesthesia may influence one or more of these forces, it is important for the anesthesiologist to know well the physiology and physiopathology of these forces. Uterine activity is defined as the product of the intensity of uterine contractions in mm Hg (measured via a catheter in the amniotic sac) multiplied by the frequency (number of contractions for 10 minutes) and expressed in mm Hg per 10 minutes, or Montevideo units. During the first 35 weeks of gestation, uterine activity is less than 20 Montevideo units and consists of one small (20 mm Hg or less) contraction every 10 minutes or more. Subsequently, these are replaced by rhythmic, coordinated contractions that increase to a frequency of 1–2 per 10 minutes and an intensity of 25-40 mm Hg. Since these stronger and slower Braxton Hicks contractions help to demarcate the uterus into upper and lower segments and cause progressive ripening and effacement of the cervix, this period is called *prelabor*.

Clinical labor is considered to have started when the cervix becomes 2–3 cm dilated and continues to dilate. During the first stages of labor, the expulsive forces are supplied solely by the contraction of the uterus. Uterine contractions are normal when there is fundal dominance, a descending gradient, an intensity of 30-60 mm Hg or more, a frequency of 3-5 per 10 minute period, and ample time for relaxation between contractions so that the resting tone is 8-12 mm Hg. The functions of these contractions is to efface and dilate the cervix and to cause progressive descent of the fetal presenting part. By plotting cervical dilation on a time ordinate, a well defined sigmoid curve is seen in normal labor (Figure 26). Two-thirds of the time of the first stage is consumed by the latent phase (which is very slow) and the other third by the active phase. In parturients who, on admission, have a cervical dilitation of less than 2 cm, the mean duration of the first stage is approximately 9 hours for primiparas and about 7 hours for multiparas. Since most parturients, on admission to the hospital, have cervical dilatation of 3 cm or more, the duration of the first stage is 6 hours or less in the primiparas and 4 hours or less in multiparas.

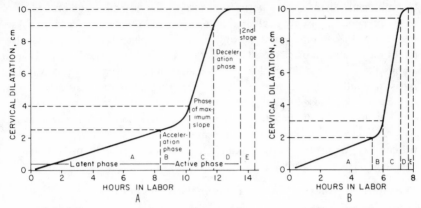

FIGURE 26. Mean labor curves of primigravidas (left) and multiparas (right). The cervical dilatation (vertical axis) is plotted against time (horizontal axis): (a) the latent phase extends from the onset of labor taken arbitrarily from the onset of regular uterine contractions to the beginning of the active phase. The onset of the active phase is apparent on the graph as that point at which the rate of dilatation (slope) begins to change, the curve becoming more steeply inclined. The active phase is divided into three phases; (b) acceleration; (c) maximum slope; and, (d) deceleration. Many obstetricians believe that the deceleration phase does not occur. The active phase ends at full dilatation giving way to the second stage of labor. (Modified from and courtesy of Friedman, E.A.: Obstet. Gynecol. 6:567, 1955.)

During the second stage of labor, uterine contractility increases further and is now aided by the auxiliary forces or bearing-down efforts of the mother—an involuntary reflex consisting of deep inspiration and the simultaneous closure of the glottis and contractions of the diaphragm and abdominal muscles. Since uterine contractility alone can produce a maximum of only 2/3rds the force necessary to expel the infant, the added force produced by the bearing-down effort is needed for spontaneous delivery. The reflex is initiated only after the cervix is completely dilated and the presenting part distends the perineum, apparently stimulating sensitive structures and thus initiating impulses that pass through the pudendal nerves and other sensory nerves supplying the perineum to the spinal cord and then ascend within the neuraxis to be integrated somewhere in the brain stem where efferent impulses originate and then are conveyed to the appropriate muscles. The duration of the second stage averages about 30–40 minutes in primiparas and 15–25 minutes in multiparas.

The progress of labor can be monitored by measuring the uterine activity, cervical dilatation, and advance of the fetal presenting part. Uterine activity can be monitored crudely by manual palpation but in many hospitals it is monitored continuously by either a pressure transducer with a sensor consisting of a fluid-filled catheter inserted into the uterine cavity and connected to the transducer, or, if the cervix is insufficiently dilated to permit the placement of such a catheter, uterine contractions can be monitored by an external transducer placed on the lower anterior abdominal wall. The changes in uterine activity are presented by both visual display and a permanent record. Cervical dilatation and advance of the presenting part are evaluated at intervals and plotted on a record. These, together with continuous monitoring of the fetal electrocardiograph and frequent measurement of maternal blood pressure, should be standard practice in all hospitals. In those hospitals where the electronic equipment is not available, measurement at regular intervals of the various parameters should be carried out. By plotting these on the "partograph," the obstetric team is able to make a rapid evaluation of the progress of labor and the dynamic aspects of the maternal and fetal condition. Numerous clinical studies have shown that the cervimetric curves and the other variables can help the obstetric team in the "active management of labor" (Figure 27).

The Effects of Drugs and Other Factors on the Forces of Labor

Large doses of sedatives and narcotics or regional analgesia or both, administered during the latent phase of the first stage retard labor, whereas, if these are given during the active phase, they have little or no effect on the progress of labor. With the parturient in the supine position, uterine contractions have a lower intensity, faster frequency, and higher tonus than when she lies on her side, sits, or squats. These are probably related to decreasing uterine blood flow. Systemic arterial hypotension frequently causes decrease in intensity and duration and impairs rhythmicity, whereas, hypertension has the opposite effects. Pain, fear, anxiety, apprehension, and other emotional reactions may impair uterine contractions. Subarachnoid and extradural block may produce a transient decrease in uterine contractility, but, if started in the active phase, labor progresses normally. It deserves emphasis that if uterine contractions are being stimulated by oxytocin or other oxytocic agents, then systemic analgesics, tranquilizers, sedatives, and regional analgesia will *not* retard the progress of labor, even when these are given in the latent phase.

The second stage of labor can be prolonged by subarachnoid and extradural block and occasionally by pudendal block because these eliminate the afferent limb of the reflex urge to bear down. This effect occurs especially if the level of analgesia is significantly above T_{10} and high concentrations are used which will produce paralysis of the lower abdominal muscles. Under such circumstances, the parturient cannot exert sufficient increase in intra-abdominal pressure to effectively help the uterus expel the infant. Moreover, if these regional procedures paralyze the perineum, the parturient looses the resistant forces and consequently internal rotation does not take place, thus increasing the incidence of persistent posterior position and the need for instrument delivery. On the other hand, if the level of analgesia does not extend above T_{10} and an optimal dose of drug is used, subarachnoid block should not impair the parturient's ability to contract the diaphragm and abdominal muscles, because the level of motor block is usually 2–3 segments below the level of analgesia. Moreover, by using low concentration of local anesthetic for epidural analgesia during the entire first stage and early second stage, the parturient maintains the ability to contract the

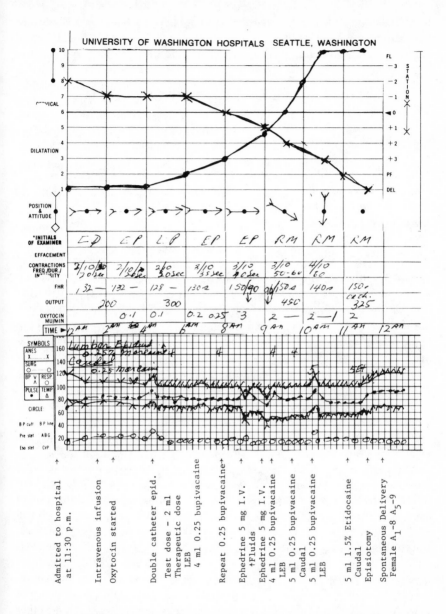

FIGURE 27. An actual partograph of primigravida (LB) managed by double catheter epidural analgesia-anesthesia. In the upper graph, the vertical axis on the left indicates cervical dilation in centimeters while on the right indiates the station of the presenting part. The lower portion contains the anesthetic record, modified, and the original handwritten remarks typed for the sake of clarity. Note bouts of mild hypertension caused by labor pain and the delivery. Two bouts of hypotension caused by supine position during examinations were unrelieved by placing the gravida on her side and late decelerations occured that were effectively treated with small doses of ephedrine.

diaphragm and abdominal muscles and will not have perineal paralysis, so that internal rotation is *not* interfered with and the parturient can delivery spontaneously by voluntarily bearing down. (See Chapter 9 and Figure 27.)

THE NATURE OF PAIN OF PARTURITION

Proper management of the parturient requires thorough knowledge of: the nature of the pain of parturition, including the mechanisms that initiate nociceptive impulses in the uterus, perineum, and pelvis; current concepts of central mechanisms involved in transmission and modulation of nociceptive information; the factors that affect the pain of childbirth; and, most importantly, the effects of parturition pain on the mother, the fetal-placental complex, the forces of labor, and the newborn.

Mechanisms of Parturition Pain

Although the exact neurophysiologic and biochemical mechanisms that produce pain during the various stages of labor and vaginal delivery have not been conclusively determined, it appears that pain is due to four factors: (a) dilatation of the cervix; (b) contraction and distension of the uterus; (c) distension of the outlet, vulva, and perineum; and (d) a heterogenous group of other factors. During the first stage, pain is due to stretching and possible tearing of the cervix and contraction and distension of the uterus. It is probable that pressure and stretch of the uterine muscles stimulate high threshold mechanical nociceptors* repeatedly and lower their thresholds. Moreover, it is possible that contractions cause cellular breakdown with the liberation of "pain producing substances" that diffuse into the extracellular space and there decrease the threshold of nociceptors. During the second stage, the stretching and actual tearing of fascia, skin, subcutaneous tissue, and other somatic structures in the perineum that are pain sensitive stimulate nociceptors in these structures. Other factors that probably contribute to the pain of childbirth include: (1) traction and pressure on the adnexa and parietal peritoneum and the structures they envelope; (2) pressure on and stretch of the bladder, urethra, rectum, and other pain-sensitive structures in the pelvis; (3) pressure on one or more roots of the lumbosacral plexus; and (4) reflex skeletal muscle spasm and vasospasm in these structures supplied by the same spinal cord segments supplying the uterus.

The nociceptive stimulation activates "bare" nerve terminals that are uniquely sensitive to noxious stimulation and are endings of subsets of the thinly myelinated A delta and the unmyelinated C fibers. Although the exact mechanisms by which noxious stimuli activate these nociceptors and cause them to transduce it into impulses is unknown, specific peptides such as bradykinin-like substances are probably involved.

---

* Nociceptors are receptors of nerve terminals that respond only to "nociceptive" or "noxious" stimulation, i.e., stimulation that is actually or potentially damaging to tissues.

Parturition Peripheral Pain Pathways

The A delta and C fibers that supply the uterus constitute visceral afferents that accompany the sympathetic nerves and pass sequentially through: (a) the uterine and cervical plexuses; (b) the pelvic (inferior hypogastric) plexus; (c) the middle hypogastric plexus or nerve; (d) the superior hypogastric plexus; and (e) thence through the lumbar and lower thoracic sympathetic chain which they leave by way of the white rami communicantes associated with the 10th, 11th, and 12th thoracic and 1st formed spinal nerves. These nociceptive afferents then pass through the posterior roots of these nerves, enter the spinal cord, and make synaptic contact with interneurons in the dorsal horn (Figure 28).

The mild pain of uterine contractions of early labor is transmitted to the 10th and 11th spinal cord segments, but, when contractions become more intense and the pain is severe, the adjacent two segments become involved. It deserves emphasis that the cervix is supplied by the same segments (T_{10}-L_1) as the body of the uterus and not through sensory nerves associated with the nervi erigentes that enter the spinal cord at S_2-S_3 and S_4 as generally believed and stated in virtually every anatomy textbook in current use. The uterine contraction pain is re-

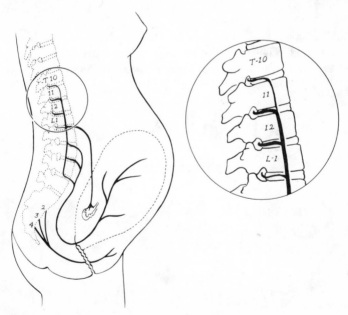

FIGURE 28. Peripheral parturition pain pathways. The uterus, including the cervix, is supplied by sensory (pain) fibers that pass from the uterus to the spinal cord by accompanying sympathetic nerves in the sequence summarized in the text. The primary pathways (shown as thick lines in the inset) enter the 11th and 12th spinal segments while the secondary auxiliary pathways enter at T_{10} and L_1. The pathways from the perineum pass to the sacral spinal cord via the pudendal nerves. (Modified from and courtesy of Bonica, J.J.: *Principles and Practice of Obstetric Analgesia and Anesthesia,* Philadelphia, F.A. Davis Company, 1967.)

ferred to the skin supplied by these four spinal segments (Figures 29a and 29b): the abdominal wall between the umbilicus and the symphysis pubis anteriorly; the skin and subcutaneous tissue over the iliac crests and upper gluteal regions laterally; and the skin and subcutaneous tissue overlying the lower four lumbar vertebrae and the upper half of the sacrum.*

The A delta and C fibers that supply the perineum and are stimulated during the second stage pass to the spinal cord primarily through the pudendal nerves

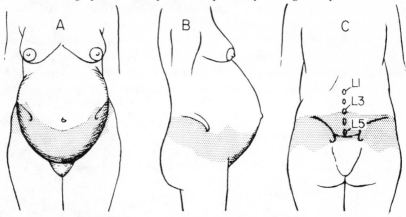

EARLY FIRST STAGE : Pain Intensity **Moderate**

FIGURE 29a. The pain associated with uterine contraction during the early part of the first stage referred to the 11th and 12th thoracic dermatomes.

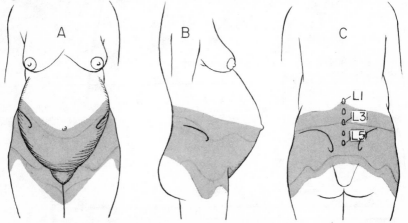

LATE FIRST STAGE : Pain Intensity Severe

FIGURE 29b. Severe pain produced by intense uterine contractions during the latter part of the first stage referred to T_{10}, T_{11}, T_{12}, and L_1 dermatomes.

---

* It should be recalled that the posterior divisions of the lower thoracic and lumbar nerves migrate caudally for a considerable distance before they emerge to supply the skin and subcutaneous tissue and adjacent paravertebral region. Thus, the cutaneous branches of the posterior division of T_{10} supply the skin at the level of the spinous processes of L_2 and L_3 vertebrae, those of T_{11} supply the skin overlying L_3 and L_4, while T_{12} supplies the skin over L_5 and S_1, and L_1 supplies those tissues over the upper part of the sacrum.

46

and make synaptic connections with interneurons of S_2, S_3, and S_4 spinal cord segments. Like other pain caused by stimulation of superficial somatic structures, the perineal pain is sharp and well localized to the perineum (Figures 30a and 30b).

The nociceptive A delta and C fibers that supply the pelvic structures that may

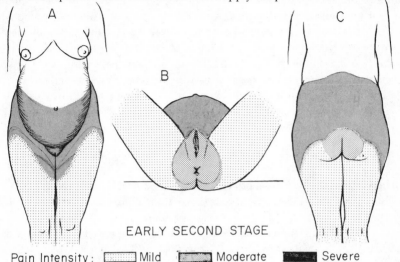

EARLY SECOND STAGE

Pain Intensity: ▭ Mild ▨ Moderate ▰ Severe

FIGURE 30a. Distribution of labor pain during the early phase of the second stage. Uterine contractions remain intense and produce severe pain in $T_{10}-L_1$ dermatomes, and, at the same time, the presenting part exerts pressure on pelvic structures and thus causes moderate pain in the very low back and perineum and often mild pain in the thighs and legs.

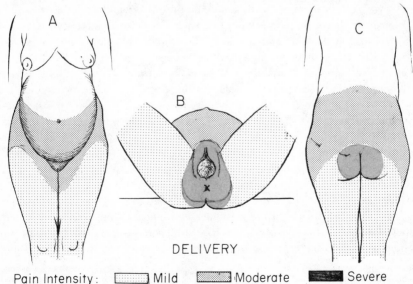

DELIVERY

Pain Intensity: ▭ Mild ▨ Moderate ▰ Severe

FIGURE 30b. Distribution of parturition pain during the latter phase of the second stage and in the actual delivery. The perineal component is the primary cause of discomfort. Uterine contractions produce moderate pain.

47

be a source of nociceptive stimulation and pain during the latter part of the first stage and during the second are components of visceral and somatic nerves that enter the spinal cord at levels T_{10}-S_5 inclusive. Nociceptive stimulation of visceral structures produces pain referred to lower thoracic and upper lumbar dermatomes; stimulation of those structures supplied by somatic nerves, including the parietal peritoneum, uterine ligaments, fascia, ligaments, and muscles of the pelvic cavity, causes pain referred to the lower lumbar and sacral segments; pressure on one or more roots of the lumbosacral plexus will cause pain referred to the back and to the back of the thighs and perhaps the legs. In patients with persistent posterior position of the presenting part or with dystocia, there is intense stimulation from uterine distension and the pelvic structures which produces severe pain in the low back and thighs. To relieve such pain, segments L_2-S_3 must be blocked.

Central Nociceptive (Pain) Mechanisms

The peripheral nociceptive afferents enter the dorsal horn of the spinal cord and synapse with large marginal cells (lamina I) that are exclusively nociceptive interneurons and also with the dendrites of neurons located predominantly in lamina V but also in laminae IV and VI. The latter group are wide dynamic range neurons that are excited by both large myelinated (A beta) low-threshold afferents and high-threshold myelinated and unmyelinated afferents. Both sets of neurons send axons which make up the spinothalamic tract predominantly contralaterally, but a few pass ipsilaterally. Moreover, these neurons make synaptic connections with interneurons that send axons to the anterior and anterolateral horn where they synapse with somatomotor and sympathetic motor neurons respectively. Particularly important in obstetric anesthesia is the fact that all of the lamina V cells that respond to visceral high-threshold afferents also respond to low-threshold cutaneous afferents from an area of skin supplied by the same spinal cord segments. Thus, these lamina V cells provide a neural basis for the phenomena of referred pain that occurs during uterine contractions (Figure 31).

The dorsal horn, which traditionally was considered as a mere transmission station, has been found to have many varieties of neurons and synaptic arrangements that permit not only reception and transmission but also a high degree of sensory processing, including local abstraction, integration, selection, and diversion of impulses. Moreover, the dorsal horn is an important site for the modulation of nociceptive information as disussed below.

After being subjected to modulating influences, some of the nociceptive impulses* from the dorsal horn pass to the anterior and anterolateral horns where they stimulate neurons whose axons constitute peripheral somatic motor nerves and sympathetic nerves, respectively, that become involved in segmental (noci-

---

* Most authorities define pain as an unpleasant perceptual and emotional experience that takes place in high cortical parts of the brain in the awake, conscious human being. Therefore, the impulses or messages produced by tissue damage are referred to as "noxious" or "nociceptive" and not "pain" during the transmission from the site of stimulation to the higher cortical center.

fensive) reflexes. Other impulses pass through the contralateral and some to the ipsilateral spinothalamic systems and other ascending pathways that convey them to the brain stem and cerebrum to provoke suprasegmental reflex responses, the perception of pain, and the three important pyschologic dimensions of pain: sensory-discriminative, motivational-affective, and cognitive-evaluative. It has been suggested that those impulses that pass cephalad via the neospinothalmic tract, the fibers of which show discrete somatotopic organization, subserve the discriminative aspects of pain and permit the organism to recognize the site, intensity, and duration of nociceptive stimulation and its physical nature (thermal, mechanical, chemical). The older palespinothalmic tract is

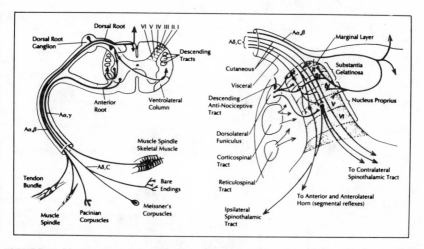

FIGURE 31. Nociceptive (and other afferent and efferent) pathways in a spinal nerve (left) and their disposition in the dorsal horn of the spinal cord (right). The large and medium size A alpha and beta afferent fibers are concerned with proprioception, touch, and pressure. The A alpha and gamma efferent fibers control reflex and skeletal muscle function while the small thinly myelinated A delta and unmyelinated C fibers transmit innocuous mechanical and thermal as well as nociceptive information. The diagram on the right shows the disposition of these and other fibers in the dorsal horn of the spinal cord in greater detail. The large tactile fibers branch into short descending and long ascending fibers that make up the dorsal columns and a lateral (recurrent) branch which send excitatory presynaptic terminals to the dendrites of deep dorsal horn neurons and to inhibitory interneurons in the substantia gelatinosa. The small A delta and C nociceptive afferents make synaptic contact with the large marginal nociceptive neurons, the axons of which pass to the contralateral side to make up the spinothalamic tract. Other A delta and C nociceptive neurons send excitatory presynaptic terminals to the dendrites of neurons in lamina V and also to neurons in laminae IV and VI. The convergence of cutaneous and visceral afferents on cells of lamina V constitute the neural basis for referred pain. Nociceptive neurons from the dorsal horn also transmit impulses to somatomotor neurons in the anterior horn and preganglionic sympathetic neurons in the anterolateral horn which become involved in segmental reflexes. The supraspinal descending tracts make connection with dorsal, ventral, and ventrolateral horn cells and modulate their output. The dorsolateral funiculus contains descendng inhibitory fibers that make contact with cells in laminae I, II, and probably V, and function to impair or block the transmission of nociceptive impulses.

composed of short fibers that project to the reticular formation, lateral pons, midbrain, and medial intralaminar thalamic nuclei and thence to the hypothalamus, limbic forebrain structures, and various parts of the cortex. This part of the system is involved in activating suprasegmental reflex response concerned with ventilation, circulation, and endocrine function, and also provokes the powerful motivational drive and unpleasant affect of pain (Figure 32).

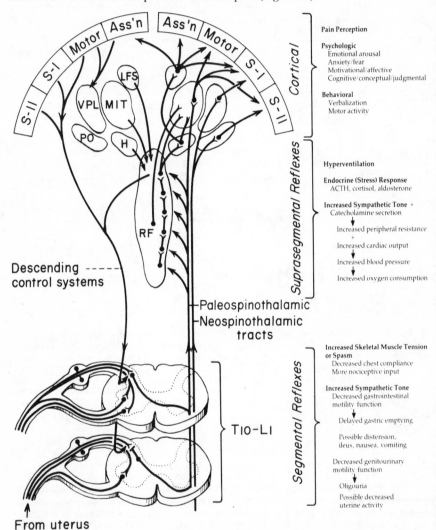

FIGURE 32. The ascending neural pathways in the neuraxis primarily involved in transmission of nociceptive information to anterior and anterolateral horn cells and to the brain and descending pathways that convey modulating influences from the brain to the spinal cord. On the right are listed segmental and suprasegmental reflex responses. Abbreviations: NGC — nucleus gigantocellularis; H — hypothalamus; PO — posterior thalamus; VPL — ventral posterolateral thalamus; MIT — medial and intralaminar thalamic nuclei; LFS — limbic forebrain structures; S_1 and S_2 — somatosensory cortex.

Modulation and Transmission of Nociceptive Information

In contrast to the older idea of straight-through transmission of nociceptive information without modification, new data make it impressively clear there is an incredible degree of modulation all along the course of transmission of noci-

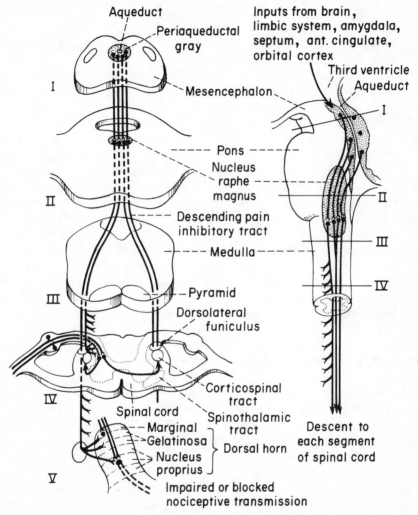

FIGURE 33. Anatomic schema of the supraspinal descending pain inhibitory system. The horizontal lines labeled I–IV indicate the levels of the cross section shown on the left while the right is a schematic sagittal section of the same structures. Neurons of the periaqueductal gray (stippled area around the aqueduct of Sylvius) send axons to the nucleus raphe magnus where they synapse with serotonergic neurons. These, in turn, send long axons descending through the medulla lateral to the pyramidal tract and through the dorsolateral funiculus of the spinal cord just lateral to the lateral corticospinal tract. Termination of these axons enter the dorsal horn at various levels of the spinal cord where they make synaptic contacts with neurons in laminae I, II, and probably V, as depicted in section IV and V of the cross sectional drawing on the left (and the right panel of Figure 31).

ceptive impulses from the uterus to the brain. In the peripheral system, the repetitive nociceptive stimulation of uterine contractions most likely lowers the threshold of nociceptors so that subsequently innocuous stimuli produce pain and associated responses. Moreover, the degree of nociceptive input from the periphery is influenced by temperature, sympathetic function, vasculature, and chemical environment of nociceptors. However, the greatest degree of modulation occurs in the dorsal horn and other parts of the central nervous system and is affected by input from different sized peripheral nerves and by local, segmental (spinal cord), and supraspinal descending influences. Modulation is achieved through the phenomena of excitation, inhibition, convergence, summation, and divergence and may have a net effect of either decreasing—and even eliminating—or increasing nociceptive transmission and, consequently, pain.

One of the most powerful descending inhibitory systems is depicted in Figure 33 and summarized in the legend. It is to be noted that activation of neurons in the periaqueductal gray (PAG) generates impulses that descend through axons that make synaptic contacts with neurons in nucleus raphe magnus, the axons of which are serotonergic and descend and make synaptic contact with terminals of primary peripheral afferents and with interneurons in laminae I, II, and V. Through these complex synaptic arrangements, they exert, either directly or through small short-axon interneurons of the substantia gelatinosa, either presynaptic inhibition of primary afferents or postsynaptic inhibition of spinothalamic neurons. Although the exact biochemical mechanism is not know, modulatory influence may be achieved through enkephalins that are released from the terminals of short axon interneurons that act as neuromodulators or as transmitters to modulate synaptic nociceptive transmission.

Factors That Influence the Pain of Childbirth

Parturients differ widely in the amount of pain and suffering they experience during childbirth, and even the same parturient has varying degrees of pain at different stages of labor and certainly during different labors. This variability is due to differences in physical factors, psychologic factors, or both.

Physical factors that influence labor pain include: (1) the intensity and duration of uterine contractions; (2) the degree of dilatation of the cervix and the speed with which this is achieved with each contraction; (3) the distension of perineal tissue; and (4) various other physical factors such as age, parity, condition of the cervix at the onset of labor, relation of the infant to the size of the birth canal, and the general condition of the parturient. Many of these factors are interrelated. For instance, an elderly primipara experiences a longer more painful labor than a young primipara. The cervix of a multipara beings to soften even before the onset of labor and is less sensitive than that of a primipara. In the presence of dystocia due to a contracted pelvis or a large baby, the gravida experiences more pain than under normal conditions. Fatigue, loss of sleep, anemia, general debility, and malnutrition exert a great influence on the patient's tolerance to the painful experience and consequently modify her behavior.

The nociceptive input coming from the periphery to the brain initiates three major **psychological dimensions**: (1) anxiety and emotional arousal; (2) motivational and affective dimensions; and (3) cognitive-conceptual-judgmental dimensions. Each of these psychologic factors can exacerbate the nociceptive input and any other of the psychologic factors. For example, the anxiety and emotional arousal stimulated by the nociceptive input through psychophysiologic mechanisms increases the skeletal muscle tension that adds to the nociceptive input and also may cause vasospasm and consequent ischemia that produces biochemical changes in tissues that lower the threshold of nociceptors. Moreover, motivational affective factors influence the degree of emotional stress and avoidance behavior manifested by an individual. The cognitive-conceptual-judgemental dimensions are influenced by the upbringing, personality, attitude, beliefs, past experience, and sociocultural factors and interpersonal transactions. Consequently, parturition pain may be influenced by any and all of these factors as well as by mentation, attitude, and the mood of the parturient at the time of labor.

It is well known that anxiety, fear and apprehension will enhance the parturient's nociceptive transmission and emotional responses to the labor pain she perceives. As mentioned in Chapter 1, one of the most frequent causes of anxiety and fear is ignorance or misinformation about the process of pregnancy and parturition and the significance of labor pain. The primigravida who has been psychologically conditioned to believe that the pain of labor augurs an event that is attendant with danger will react differently from the well informed parturient who has been adequately prepared. Inappropriate remarks or words may prove strong "negative" suggestions to the end that sensations are intensified and pain becomes exaggerated. Finally, many cultural patterns and customs are conducive to overt expression of pain and suffering.

Suggestion, distraction, and motivation are highly effective in modulating (inhibiting) nociceptive transmission and the affective dimensions of pain. They are inextricably interrelated with the amount of confidence the parturient has in her physician or midwife and the understanding or feelings she has about the process of childbirth. It has been shown conclusively that prenatal education of the gravida often decreases or eliminates anxiety, fear, and apprehension, and may initiate psychodynamic mechanisms that actually diminish transmission of nociceptive information.

The aforementioned recent data about supraspinal descending influences explain how psychologic factors can increase or decrease the labor pain. On one hand, emotional, motivational, and affective factors promptly activate the cortical mechanisms in the brain that may stimulate periaqueductal neurons and thus increase the activity of the aforementioned supraspinal descending inhibitory system that prevents or impairs the transmission of nociceptive information in the dorsal horn and in different levels of the neuraxis. On the other hand, under appropriate conditions, anxiety, fear, and apprehension may activate certain brain mechanisms that inhibit the efficacy of supraspinal descending inhibitory systems that, in turn, enhance the transmission of nociceptive impulses, resulting in greater pain perception that, in turn, may increase the anxiety, fear, and emotional arousal. Thus a "vicious circle" is initiated and will persist unless it is interrupted by psychologic and pharmacologic procedures.

Summary

It appears that the pain and associated responses to noxious stimulation provoked by uterine contractions and other tissue damaging factors are the net effects of highly complex interactions of various neural systems, modulating influences, and psychologic factors. Through the interaction of the afferent systems and neocortical processes, the individual is provided perceptual and discriminative information that is analyzed and that usually activates motivational and cognitive processes. These, in turn, act on the motor system and initiate psychodynamic mechanisms that produce complex physiologic, behavioral, and affective responses that characterize acute pain. In general, the immediate responses to the nociceptive stimulation consist of: (1) involuntary (automatic) responses involving segmental and suprasegmental reflex mechanisms normally intended to preserve homeostasis and mainifested by contraction or spasm of skeletal muscles, vasoconstriction, cardiovascular and ventilatory changes, alterations of other visceral changes, alterations of other visceral functions, and widespread endocrine respones; and (2) cerebral cortical responses that include (a) the emotional experience we call pain, (b) affective reaction of anxiety and apprehension, and (c) operant responses characteristic of overt pain behavior such as verbalization, screaming or moaning, grimacing, posturing, prompt withdrawal of the injured part, or a combination of all these.

DELETERIOUS EFFECTS OF PARTURITION PAIN

From time immemorial it has been universally appreciated that the pain of uterine contractions has the important biological function of signalling the onset of labor. Moreover, in the last half century it has been recognized that the physiologic, biochemical, and psychologic responses are intended to preserve homeostasis. Many proponents of natural childbirth claim that the experience of the pain is a part of the normal delivery process and is essential to the emotional well-being of the mother and the normal psychologic and physiologic development of the baby. However, what has not been realized is that, if labor pain is not relieved when it becomes severe, it is likely to have deleterious effects on the mother, fetus, and newborn. The persistent pain and stress enhance the segmental and suprasegmental reflex responses that then become abnormal and cause exaggerated effects on ventilation, circulation, endocrine function, and

54

other body functions. Although these have been alluded to in Chapter 1, they are reemphasized here.

Human studies in unpremedicated primigravidas in labor have shown that the pain of uterine contractions causes a fivefold to twentyfold increase in ventilation with consequent severe respiratory alkalosis, a significant increase in sympathetic activity and norepinephrine release that causes a 50–150% increase in cardiac output, a 20–40% increase in blood pressure, and significant increases in metabolism and oxygen consumption, and decreases in gastrointestinal and urinary bladder motility, and, at times, in uterine contractility. The increased load on the heart and circulation is tolerated well by a healthy gravida but may prove deleterious to parturients with heart disease. The increase in oxygen consumption caused by the pain and work of labor, together with the loss of bicarbonate from the kidney as compensation for the respiratory alkalosis, and often reduction in carbohydrate intake, usually produce a progressive metabolic acidosis that not only is deleterious to the mother but is also transferred to the fetus. Some have suggested that this is due, in part, to pain-induced reflex vasoconstriction of peripheral tissue with consequent inadequate perfusion and hypoxia. Finally, the decrease in gastrointestinal motility causes retention of fluid and food in the stomach and increases the risk of aspiration of gastric contents.

Pain induced in pregnant baboons, ewes, and other animals produces a significant (25–35%) increase in catecholamines, particularly norepinephrine, with a consequent 35–70% decrease in uterine blood flow (Figure 34). These effects

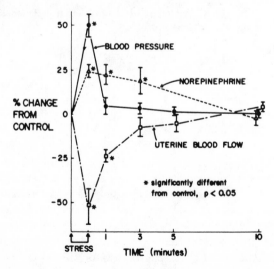

FIGURE 34. The effects of pain-induced stress on maternal arterial blood pressure, noradrenalin blood level, and uterine blood flow. The stress was induced by application of an electric current on the skin of a ewe at term. Note that the increase in arterial pressure is very transient but the decay in norepinephrine level is more protracted and is reflected by a mirror-image decrease in uterine blood flow. (Courtesy of Shnider, S.M., et al.: Anesthesiology 50:30, 1979.)

were also noted in animals subjected to fear and psychologic stress (Figure 35). Moreover, it has been found that severe pain and anxiety during human labor causes an increase in norepinephrine and epinephrine which was attenuated significantly after institution of regional analgesia. Severe hyperventilation with consequent severe respiratory alkalosis causes a shift in the maternal oxygen dissociation curve that impairs the transfer of oxygen to the fetus. This effect, together with the reduction in uterine blood flow provoked by the increased norepinephrine release, is likely to further impair placental blood gas exchange. The incidence of such series of intermittent impairment of placental blood gas exchange is apparently tolerated by the normal fetus, but, if the fetus is already

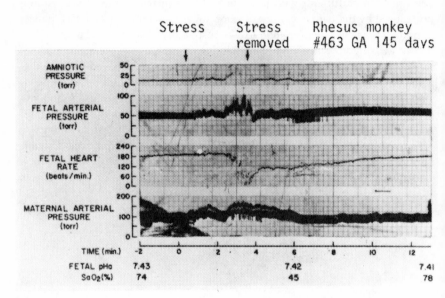

FIGURE 35. Effects of pain-induced stress on maternal arterial pressure, intrauterine pressure, and fetal heart rate in a pregnant monkey. Note the adverse effect of the stress on fetal heart rate and oxygenation. (Modified from and courtesy of Morishima, et al.: Am. J. Obstet. Gynecol. 131:286, 1978.)

at risk because of obstetric complications, the pain-induced reduction of oxygen may be the critical factor that produces morbidity or even mortality.

In addition to the significant increase in plasma catecholamines provoked by the pain of labor, there is an elevation of plasma corticosteriods, and maternal ACTH and cortisol levels rise as labor progresses, reaching maximum values immediately prior to the delivery. The pain and stress also increase the secretion of free fatty acids and other endocrines that may have deleterious effects on the mother and fetus. Partial relief of pain with systemic analgesics decreases the degree of endocrine response, while continuous epidural analgesia prevents it entirely.

CHAPTER 4. PHARMACOLOGY OF OBSTETRIC ANALGESICS, ANESTHETICS, AND RELATED DRUGS

Currently, many drugs and techniques are available to provide relief of childbirth pain. The methods vary from one area to another and from one country to another, depending upon the culture, medical personnel, facilities, and many other sociologic and professional factors. For proper clinical application, each of these drugs and techniques must be evaluated from five interrelated viewpoints: (1) analgesic potency or other therapeutic efficacy; (2) side effects on the mother; (3) side effects on the fetus; (4) residual effects on the newborn; and (5) side effects on labor. Table 4 contains a critical evaluation of the drugs and techniques in common use from these five viewpoints. Although some drugs, such as the barbiturates, scopolamine, and the inhalation agents, cyclopropane and diethyl ether, are no longer used in most obstetric centers, they are included in this table for the information of those that may still be using them.

The effects on the mother, fetus and newborn, and the force of labor listed in the table are based on the use of optimal doses (OD) and optimal route of administration of systemic drugs and the use of optimal concentrations and volumes of local anesthetics as listed in Table 10, page 88. The effects on the newborn are based on clinical evaluation by the Apgar Score, acid-base status, electronic monitoring during labor, and the recent use of Early Neonatal Neurobehavioral Scale (ENNS). For example, administration of epidural analgesia with 12–15 ml of 1.5–2% lidocaine or mepivacaine is associated with neonatal depression assessed by ENNS, whereas, 0.5% bupivacaine is not. However, since 0.5–0.75% lidocaine or mepivacaine is adequate for obstetric analgesia, it is likely to result in less or no neonatal depression. Similarly, the use of single doses of 2 mg/kg thiopental for induction of balanced anesthesia for cesarean section does not produce low ENNS scores, whereas, doses of 4 mg/kg or greater do. Moreover, in applying this information to a particular patient, it is important to realize that these effects are modified by the changes produced by pregnancy and labor and the pathophysiology of any obstetric or medical complication present. Comments to emphasize the most important aspects of each of these agents when used for different obstetric indications will be made subsequently.

TABLE 4. PHARMACOLOGY OF OBSTETRIC ANALGESIA-ANESTHESIA (PART A)

| | SEDATIVES/TRANQUILIZERS | | | | ANALGESICS |
	A	B	C	D	E
Specific Drugs	Promazine Hydroxyzine	Diazepam (Valium)	Scopolamine	Secobarbital Pentobarbital	Meperidine (Demerol (D), Pethidine) Morphine (M) Pentazocine (P) (Talwin)
Optimal Dose and Route	50 mg IM	5–10 mg IV	0.3–0.6 mg PO	100 mg PO	D—100 mg IM M—10 mg IM P —50 mg IM or ½ dose IV **slowly**
Therapeutic Effects	Sedation, decrease of anxiety; Antiemetic	Sedation, tranquility, some amnesia	Amnesia, sedation	Sedation, induces sleep	Analgesia, sedation, and decrease of anxiety due to pain relief
Side Effects on Mother	None	↓ Respiration between contractions	Some disorientation; CNS ↓ when combined with barbiturates	None with OD; Depression with overdose	↓ Respiration between contractions; delayed gastric emptying; nausea and vomiting in some
Effects on Labor	None	None	None	None	None
Placental Transfer		**Rapid** Within 3–5 minutes after IM or 60 seconds after IV			Same as A
Effects on Fetus	Slight **CNS** ↓* ↓ BBV**	**CNS** ↓ ↓ BBV	Slight **CNS** ↓	Some **CNS** ↓ ↓ BBV	Moderate **CNS** ↓ and **CV** ↓ ↓ BBV
Effects on Newborn	Slight respiratory ↓	Neonatal ↓ hypotonia ↓ EEG, ENNS, ↓ thermo-regulation	Not studied	Mild ↓ ↓ EEG, ENNS	moderate **CNS** ↓ ↓ EEG, ENNS
Remarks	Used alone during latent phase and combined with narcotics during active phase	Potent sedative and tranquilizer, but side effects on fetus and newborn	No longer widely used	No longer used except early latent phase to induce sleep	Effective analgesics for moderate pain in 70–80% of parturients

*↓ = depression of   **↓ BBV = decrease or loss of beat-to-beat variability   CNS = central nervous system; CV = cardiovascular; ENNS = Early Neonatal Neurobehavioral Scale; IM = intramuscular; IV = intravenous; PO = by mouth

TABLE 4. PHARMACOLOGY OF OBSTETRIC ANALGESIA-ANESTHESIA (PART B)

	REGIONAL ANALGESIA-ANESTHESIA			
	A	B	C	D
Specific Techniques	Spinal Epidural block Standard $T_{10} - S_5$ Segmental $T_{10} - L_1$ Double catheter	Caudal block (catheter tip at S_1)	Subarachnoid block (SAB) **STB**** $T_{10} - S_5$ **SB***** $S_1 - S_5$	Paracervical (PCB) Pudendal block (PB)
Therapeutic Efficacy	Greater degree of pain relief than with other regional techniques	Excellent pain relief	**STB**—analgesia for labor and delivery **SB**—anesthesia for delivery only	**PCB**—for relief of uterine pain **PB**—for relief of perineal pain
Side Effects on Mother	Minimal hypotension with proper management; moderate/severe hypotension in supine position	More hypotension than A	**STB**—more hypotension than A, B **SB**—none	None if properly done, but sedation and toxic reaction with overdose
Effects on Labor	None. If initiated too early → prolonged latent phase. This obviated with oxytocin; bearing-down reflex lost, but able to push voluntarily	Same as A	**STB**—same as A **SB**—none except loss of bearing-down reflex	**PCB**—transient depression of contractions, but no effect on labor progress **PB**—none
Placental Transfer	**Rapid** but small amounts with AC/LA*	**Rapid** but more amounts than A	None	**PCB**—rapid and more than A, B **PB**—less than A, B, or PC
Effects on Fetus	Transient ↓ BBV with lidocaine (L) and mepivacaine (MP), but none with bupivacaine (B)	Same as A but greater effects	**STB**—none unless severe and sustained hypotension → fetal distress **SB**—none	**PCB**—bradycardia ↓ BBV **PB**—same as A
Effects on Newborn	↓ENNS with 1.5–2% L or MP, but none with AC/LA, none with B	Same as A but greater degree (more LA used)	None except if severe and sustained hypotension → neonatal ↓	**PCB**— ↓ ENNS **PB**—same as A
Remarks	Excellent analgesia, but premature block of lower limbs and perineum with standard; sometimes inadequate perineal block with segmental; double catheter best technique	Same as A plus greater perineal and limb paralysis	Simple and rapid analgesia and perineal relaxation, but premature perineal and limb paralysis and loss of reflex	**PCB** plus **PB**— good analgesia; can be done by obstetrician; no hypotension

* AC/LA = analgesic concentrations (AC) of local anesthetics (LA) ** STB = standard subarachnoid block *** SB = true saddle block (For other abbreviations see Table 3, Part A)

TABLE 4. PHARMACOLOGY OF OBSTETRIC ANALGESIA-ANESTHESIA (PART C)

| | GENERAL ANALGESIA-ANESTHESIA | | |
	A	B	C
Specific Techniques	Inhalation Analgesia	Inhalation Anesthesia	Balanced Anesthesia
Specific Drugs	40–50% nitrous oxide (N_2O) 0.35% methoxyflurane (M) 0.35–0.5% trichloroethylene (TC) 3–5% cyclopropane (C) 1–1.5% diethyl ether (DE) 0.25–1.25% enflurane (E) ketamine 0.5 mg/kg	0.4–0.8% methoxyflurane 0.5–1.0% halothane (H) 0.5–1.0% enflurane 5–12% cyclopropane 2–5% diethyl ether	100% O_2 for 5 minutes 3 mg d-tubocurarine or 1 mg pancuronium → Ketamine 0.4–0.5 mg/kg and thiopental 3 mg/kg → immediate cricoid pressure → 100 mg succinylcholine (SC) IV → tracheal intubation →40% N_2O + 0.5% H in O_2 + SC infusion until delivery → increase to 60% N_2O + 0.5% H in O_2 after delivery
Therapeutic Efficacy	Satisfactory analgesia in 60–70% with N_2O, M, C, TC, and DE, 80% with E, and 90% with combination M and N_2O	Anesthesia for vaginal delivery or cesarean section; higher concentrations needed for induction	Insures adequate oxygenation, anesthesia, relaxation, and satisfactory maintenance
Side Effects on Mother	None with analgesic concentration except occasional amnesia and confusion	Slight ↓ cardiac output (CO) and blood pressure (BP) with M and H ↑ CO and BP ⎱ C, DE ↓ respiration ⎰	Respiratory depression and paralysis; artificial ventilation required
Effects on Labor	None	None with light concentrations of N_2O, M, E, and C; myometrial ↓ with H, DE	None
Placental Transfer	Rapid	Rapid	IV and inhalation agents rapid; muscle relaxants little or none
Effects on Fetus	None	↓ CNS ↓ ENNS ↓ EEG	Same as A
Effects on Newborn	None or slight neonatal ↓	Slight to moderate neonatal ↓ that can be rapidly eliminated by administering 100% O_2	None with above amounts and concentrations, moderate ↓ with larger amounts or concentrations
Remarks	C and DE no longer used, other agents provide satisfactory analgesia and are simple to administer	C and DE no longer used, others produce good general anesthesia with little or no side effects except those noted above	Best method of anesthesia in hypovolemic/ hypotensive parturients; excellent for cesarean section and for instrumental vaginal delivery

(For abbreviations see Part A)

PART B. ANALGESIA—ANESTHESIA FOR VAGINAL DELIVERY

CHAPTER 5. GENERAL CLINICAL CONSIDERATIONS

This chapter contains a brief discussion of general clinical aspects of obstetric analgesia and anesthesia that apply to all parturients regardless of the method of pain relief used. These are presented here to obviate the need of repeating them in subsequent chapters and include: (1) basic principles; (2) antepartal preparation; (3) preanesthetic care; (4) intrapartal and intra-anesthetic care; and (5) postanesthetic care. At the end of this chapter there is a table that gives an overview of various methods of analgesia and anesthesia (Table 6, p. 66).

METHODS OF OBSTETRIC ANALGESIA AND ANESTHESIA

Currently, many methods are available to provide relief of childbirth pain, including psychologic techniques and a great variety of drugs used for regional or general anesthesia. The methods used vary from one area to another and from one country to another, depending upon the culture, medical personnel available, facilities, and many other sociologic and professional factors. The many agents and techniques that are being used can arbitrarily be included in five categories which are summarized in Table 6, p. 66. It is to be noted that the table summarizes in a general way the degree of pain usually experienced by the 'average' parturient during pregnancy and various stages and phases of labor and the appropriate time for the application of the various methods to relieve it.

The table suggests that the management of the gravida during pregnancy and during the latent phase of the first stage of labor is similar, regardless of the three methods of pharmacological (chemical) analgesia-anesthesia used later on when pain becomes moderate to severe. This section will also include a brief discussion of the proper application of narcotics and other systemic analgesics except the inhalation agents.

Details of the technical aspects and management of the patient with each of the currently used agents and techniques are given in the chapters that follow. The table is presented merely to give the reader an overview and may contain suggestions regarding dose of specific drugs and time of administration that may differ from that of other writers. Moreover, it deserves re-emphasis that each of these methods has its own specific indications and that the advantages, disadvantages, and limitations of each method vary under different conditions. Proper application requires that the anesthetist and the physician or midwife delivering the patient fully appreciate this.

BASIC PRINCIPLES

To obtain best results with obstetric analgesia and anesthesia, it is essential for the obstetric team to adhere to certain basic principles. The objective is to provide optimal relief of pain to the mother without unusual risk to her or her infant. The *sine qua non* of obstetric anesthesia should always be safety for mother and child. It is the primary mission of the anesthetist to select indicated agents and techniques and employ them in such a manner as to cause the least degree of disturbance to the bodily functions of the mother and none to those of the infant. How effectively such a grave responsibility is discharged depends primarily upon the anesthetist's knowledge, judgment, skill, and experience: these are far more important than the specific drug or technique used.

Currently there is no analgesic agent or technique that offers such superior advantages over others that it can or should be used in all cases. Therefore, the patient should *never* be forced to accept a method unless unusual circumstances exist that preclude the use of all other methods. The type of analgesia and anesthesia must be tailored to the needs of the individual patient. There are many factors that must be considered in the selection of methods that will provide the best results: (1) the physiological status, psychological makeup, and the desires of the mother; (2) the condition of the fetus at the time of delivery; (3) the obstetric requirements for the delivery; (4) whether complications exist; (5) the personality, experience, skill, and practices of the physician or midwife who is to perform the delivery, as well as his or her concepts concerning obstetric analgesia-anesthesia; and (6) most importantly, the competence and skill of the anesthetist as well as the facilities that are available.

It is obvious that high quality analgesia and anesthesia require observance of the five cardinal C's—communication, coordination, cooperation, courtesy, and (sometimes) compromise by every member of the obstetric team. It is essential for the obstetrician to know well and to appreciate the advantages, disadvantages, and limitations of each method of analgesia and anesthesia so that he may integrate his management with that of the anesthetist.

ANTEPARTAL PREPARATION

One of the most basic considerations in obstetric analgesia and anesthesia is the proper mental, psychologic, and physiologic preparation of the gravida. It is generally acknowledged that the pregnant patient of today deserves and will reap great benefits from the time and effort spent by her physician in informing her (and her husband) about the course of pregnancy. This can be accomplished during the prenatal visits to the office or it can be done by having monthly group-information periods. During these periods, information is disseminated verbally and with such aides as slides, video tapes, motion pictures, manikins, and charts. The topics to be covered are the same as those listed in the next chapter (Table 7, page 73). Understanding the changes in circulation, respiration, and other systems and the alteration in endocrine function will help the gravida understand and accept the inconveniences, discomforts, and awkwardness of the lopsided silhouette she develops during pregnancy. A discussion of the physiology and clinical course of labor will similarly provide her with useful information and will help her to cooperate during labor. The procedures she is to follow during labor and delivery should be explained in detail, with the emphasis placed on the importance of properly bearing down during the second stage (in order to provide the uterus with the assistance of the auxiliary powers of labor) and of relaxing between contractions. This form of education and information is of inestimable value in freeing the expectant mother from misconceptions, superstitions, false beliefs, and fears that may have been instilled in her by misinformed relatives and friends or by improper teachings. Most important in the mental preparation of the gravida is the physician's or midwife's manifestation of friendship and sympathetic understanding, his or her kindness and reassurance, and those other human qualities that comprise the "art" of medicine and enhance the development of rapport. An optimal relationship between health worker and patient is a potent force in relieving pain and enhancing the action of analgesics.

During one of these prenatal visits, analgesia and anesthesia should be discussed in some detail and the advantages, disadvantages, and limitations of each technique should be briefly described. Although the obstetrician may indicate which technique he or she considers preferable, great caution should be exercised not to promise the patient either a specific method or painless labor. Rather, the patient should be assured that there are many means available for relieving pain and that all efforts compatible with safety will be made to lessen the discomfort. In hospitals that have complete anesthesia service, it is useful for a member of the obstetric anesthesia service to meet with groups of gravidas for periods of 60–90 minutes to discuss analgesia-anesthesia in some detail. For this purpose, the outline in Table 5 is recommended.

If the patient is to deliver in the hospital, it is essential that everyone who will come in contact with the patient (from the admission clerk to members of the house staff) be inculcated with the importance of a friendly, reassuring attitude. The obstetric nurse or midwife, by the very nature of her work and her close association with the patient during the most emotionally critical phase of the pregnancy, holds the key to either success or failure for this entire program. A warm, sympathetic attitude, reassurance, and prompt response to requests, together with the efficient discharge of the physician's orders, will do a great deal to allay fears, instill confidence, and consequently enhance the objectives of analgesia.

The gravida should be specifically instructed to refrain from eating solid foods after labor begins. It will prove profitable to explain to her that labor and medication markedly interfere with digestion and absorption and delay gastric emptying to such an extent that partially digested food may remain in the stomach for

TABLE 5. GROUP SESSION ON ANALGESIA-ANESTHESIA
(Time: 90 minutes)

I. Introduction
  A. Purpose of session
  B. Format and time schedule
II. History of Obstetric Anesthesia (5 minutes)
  A. Anesthesia in ancient times
  B. Discovery of anesthesia
  C. First use of obstetric anesthesia
  D. Queen Victoria's role in popularizing anesthesia
  E. Subsequent developments
  F. Recent advances
III. Classification of Anesthesia (25 minutes)
  A. Psychologic analgesia
    1. Hypnosis ⎫ mechanisms
    2. Natural childbirth ⎬ advantages
    3. Psychoprophylaxis ⎭ limitations
  B. General anesthesia
    1. Inhalation ⎫ brief description
    2. Intravenous ⎬ of technique advantages
    3. Rectal ⎭ limitations

C. Regional anesthesia
  1. Mechanisms ⎫
  2. Subarachnoid block ⎪ brief
  3. Extradural block ⎬ description
  4. Paracervical block ⎪ of technique
  5. Pudendal block ⎪ advantages
  6. Other ⎭ limitations
IV. General Principles of Application (15 minutes)
  A. Preanesthetic evaluation and preparation
  B. Selection of analgesia-anesthesia
    1. Factors to be considered
    2. Need to postpone selection until parturition
  C. Cooperation of gravida
V. Question and Answer Period (15–30 minutes)
VI. Informal Session (rest of period)
  A. Coffee and refreshments
  B. Informal group discussion
  C. Opportunity to ask questions privately
  D. Inspection of equipment

as long as 24 hours. Aspiration of gastric contents is currently the most frequent cause of maternal death in most parts of the world. The importance of lying on her side to avoid aortocaval compression during the last 12 weeks of pregnancy and during labor is emphasized.

PREANESTHETIC CARE

If the supplemental analgesia and subsequent anesthesia for vaginal delivery is to be administered by someone other than the attending obstetrician or midwife, it is essential that the anesthetist participate actively in preanesthetic and postanesthetic care as well as management during the anesthesia. The preanesthetic visit by the anesthetist is as important, if not more important, for obstetric patients than for surgical patients. During such a visit, the anesthetist: (1) establishes rapport with, and instills confidence in, the parturient; (2) becomes familiar with the patient's medical and anesthesia history, physical findings, and obstetric conditions; (3) evaluates the physiologic and emotional status of the parturient; (4) discusses the plans with both the obstetrician and the parturient and makes arrangements for analgesia and anesthesia; and (5) participates actively in the psychologic preparation of the gravida. She should be asked what drugs she has taken during pregnancy and if she has had any drug reactions, allergy, or other abnormal response to previous therapy. The *anesthesia history* should include details about her previous experience with anesthetics and how she feels about them. Since most patients have a subconscious fear of death, the anesthetist should make a point of emphasizing the safety of modern anesthesia.

A *physical examination* should be performed by the anesthetist not only to obtain additional information, but also to enhance rapport, for it manifests interest and concern for the patient's welfare. In gravidas who are beyond the 34th week of gestation, the blood pressure and pulse must be measured with the patient in the lateral position and again at 1, 2, and 5 minutes in the supine position, to ascertain the degree of compression of the inferior vena cava and aorta by the uterus. This maneuver will help detect severe aortocaval compession. The patient should again be impressed with the importance of lying on her side during the entire labor.

INTRAPARTAL AND INTRAANESTHETIC CARE

During labor, the uterine contractions, cervical dilatation, and advance of the presenting part should be monitored. The cervicographic method of following the progress of labor is recommended. In home deliveries and in hospital deliveries where modern equipment is not available, the fetal heart rate (FHR) is followed by auscultation. The limitations of this method and of palpating uterine contractions are generally recognized and emphasize the need for the clinical use of more sophisticated systems, especially in monitoring the labor of women with high-risk pregnancies. Currently, there are a number of systems that permit the continuous and simultaneous measurements of FHR and myometrial activity that are simple to operate, easy to maintain, and of reasonable cost. Combined with these is the measurement of the cervical dilatation and advance of the presenting part. These are recorded on a partograph which also has space for recording maternal blood pressure, respiration, the administration of oxytocins, sedatives, systemic analgesics and regional analgesia techniques, and other drugs used during labor and delivery. (See Figure 27, p. 43). In many centers, facilities are also available for assessment of pH and other biochemical parameters of the fetal blood obtained from the scalp or the buttocks. In normal uncomplicated labor, FHR varies between 120 and 160 beats/min, while the pH is 7.25 or greater.

During labor the patient is made to lie on her side and only assume the supine position for brief periods (seconds), during which left lateral tilt or left uterine displacement is used. The induction of regional analgesia is also carried out with the parturient on her side or left lateral tilt. To prevent unilateral block, the parturient is made to change sides 3–4 minutes after the initial injection. An alternative is to inject the local anesthesic solution with the parturient supine but with a wedge under her right upper thigh and gluteal region and if necessary to provide manual displacement of the uterus to prevent aortocaval compression.

TABLE 6. SUMMARY OF OBSTETRIC ANALGESIA-ANESTHESIA TECHNIQUES

PHASE OF PREGNANCY	DEGREE OF DISCOMFORT	PSYCHOLOGIC ANALGESIA EDUCATED CHILDBIRTH, HYPNOSIS
PREGNANCY	Emotional reactions Mild discomfort	Intense preparation for psychological analgesia
PARTURITION **First Stage**		
a. **Latent Phase** Onset of labor progresses to 3-cm cervical dilatation	Usually mild pain Unprepared patient has fear and anxiety, may complain of moderate or severe 'pain'	Reinforce psychologic analgesia Sedative may be needed
b. **Active Phase** Cervical dilatation (centimeters) 4	Moderate uterine pain	Reinforce psychologic analgesia
5		
6 progresses to 7 8 9	Progresses to severe pain	Narcotic often needed but in smaller doses than with other methods
10 Complete dilatation	Severe uterine pain	Continue to reinforce psychologic analgesia (plus repeat narcotics?)
Second Stage a. **Early**	Moderate perineal and other pain	Reinforce above
b. **Delivery** Spontaneous or Forceps	Severe perineal pain Perineal relaxation required	Perineal anesthesia with pudendal block desirable
Third Stage a. **Delivery of placenta** b. **Perineal repair**	Minimal uterine pain Perineal analgesia required	Maintain perineal analgesia
Fourth Stage	Little or no discomfort	

TABLE 6. SUMMARY OF OBSTETRIC ANALGESIA-ANESTHESIA TECHNIQUES (Continued)

TECHNIQUES OF PHARMACOLOGIC ANALGESIA-ANESTHESIA

SIMPLE METHODS OF ANALGESIA-ANESTHESIA	INHALATION ANALGESIA-ANESTHESIA	REGIONAL ANALGESIA-ANESTHESIA

Psychologic preparation of the gravida. Inform patient about various types of analgesia-anesthesia. Reassure about proper selection of best method. Instruct how to bear down. Request not to imbibe or eat promptly after labor begins

Good nursing care—avoid food and fluids
Psychologic support—reassurance, sympathy, suggestion, information, companionship
Pharmacologic sedation:
1. Sedatives (e.g., promethazine 50 mg IM)
2. Repeat in 1 or 2 hours
3. Give small dose of narcotic only if discomfort is severe or latent phase prolonged
4. If admitted in evening and progress slow, give 100 mg barbiturate by mouth to assure sleep. If moderate discomfort present, also give morphine 10 mg subcutaneously

SIMPLE METHODS OF ANALGESIA-ANESTHESIA	INHALATION ANALGESIA-ANESTHESIA	REGIONAL ANALGESIA-ANESTHESIA
Narcotic or Narcotic sedative } IMq 2–4 hours or IVq 1–2 hours or continuous infusion	Narcotic alone or in combination as described in column on left	Continuous extradural analgesia or subarachnoid block initiated when proper obstetric conditions prevail
Paracervical block or inhalation analgesia initiated and continued until delivery	Inhalation analgesia initiated and continued until delivery	Repeat injections to provide continuous uterine pain relief ↓ Supplement regional analgesia with small doses of narcotics or sedatives *only* if necessary
Pudendal block initiated		Perineal analgesia required: a. Extend segmental epidural, or b. Repeat caudal, or c. Initiate low caudal (double catheter), or d. Repeat spinal if necessary
Perineal anesthesia continued	Inhalation anesthesia or Balanced anesthesia	Perineal relaxation produced with high concentration of local anesthetics
	Lighten anesthesia	Maintain perineal anesthesia
	Emergence from anesthesia	Remove catheter

During the immediate preanesthetic period, the patient is reassured, informed in detail of what procedures are to be done, and given psychological support in every other way. The maternal blood pressure, pulse, respiration, and other vital signs, and the fetal heart rate are measured and recorded at frequent intervals. It is also advisable to have continuous electrocardiogram recording. In high risk patients, central venous pressure should be used to measure the load on the right atrium, and in patients with cardiovascular disease, a Swan-Ganz catheter is employed.

Maternal ventilation can be evaluated by arterial blood gas analysis, by end-expiratory carbon dioxide determination, or by measuring tidal and minute volumes clinically with the help of a Wright Respirometer. A Block-Aid Monitor will enable accurate assessment of the amount of relaxant needed in ill patients and provide essential background for their reversal. The venous hematocrit and the level of serum electrolytes should be determined on admission and repeated as indicated. Urinalysis at regular intervals is mandatory in patients suffering from metabolic disorders and during prolonged labor.

POSTANESTHETIC CARE

Total anesthetic care requires that the anesthetist care for the patient during the immediate postanesthetic period and visit her at least once daily, or more frequently, until she is discharged from the hosptial. The anesthetist should play an active role in treating postoperative pain and postpuncture headaches and in carrying out other procedures that prevent pulmonary complications.

CHAPTER 6. NONPHARMACOLOGIC METHODS OF OBSTETRIC ANALGESIA

During the past three decades there has been a progressive increase in interest and in the application of several methods that do not entail the use of pharmacologic agents to relieve the pain of childbirth. These include "natural childbirth," proposed and practiced by the late Dick-Read; the method of "psychoprophylaxis," originated by Russian physicians in the late 1940s (and soon thereafter practiced and advocated by Lamaze and colleagues in Paris and during the last quarter-century practiced world-wide); hypnosis, which has been used sporadically in a few obstetric clinics; and acupuncture and transcutaneous electrical nerve stimulation (TENS) (both of which have been given clinical trial during the past decade). This chapter will briefly describe the advantages, disadvantages, and limitations of each of these methods and will summarize the techniques used. The first three methods are considered under the term "psychologic analgesia," because, despite the claim to the contrary by their proponents, each of the methods has psychologic and neurophysiologic bases similar to the other two.

PSYCHOLOGIC ANALGESIA

Dick-Read, Lamaze, and other early proponents of natural childbirth, psychoprophylaxis, and hypnosis extolled their virtues, which included not only analgesia but shorter labors and better condition of the mother and the newborn. They insisted that with proper preparation of the gravida, childbirth was painless. Indeed, Dick-Read claimed that pain was the product of civilization and was induced by fear and tension that could be precluded with antepartal preparation and intrapartal care. Moreover, despite the general consensus among the Russian originators of psychoprophylaxis that the percentage of truly painless parturition was low, Lamaze, as late as 1959, insisted on calling it "childbirth without pain." Although data from controlled studies are meager, the available evidence suggests that, if each method is properly applied in a large group of unselected parturients, it can be expected that: (a) 10–15% will experience no pain and will require no chemical analgesia or anesthesia during parturition; (b) in an additional 20–30%, the amount of pain is diminished to varying degrees so that these parturients will require less drug-induced analgesia than unprepared paturients; and (c) in the rest, pain will not be influenced, but fear, anxiety, and apprehension will be less, and most of the gravidas will be able to be more cooperative and to participate actively in the parturition. Moreover, if each method is applied in selected parturients by zealous, well prepared physicians and health professionals, the incidence of satisfactory analgesia is further increased. These figures compare with 70–80% satisfactory (albeit not complete) analgesia obtained with narcotics, with 60–80% satisfactory analgesia obtained with an inhalation agent (used in analgesic, not anesthetic, concentrations), and with 90–95% satisfactory analgesia achieved with regional techniques properly applied.

Natural childbirth, psychoprophylaxis, and hypnosis have the following disadvantages: (a) true analgesia (complete pain relief) occurs in only a small percentage of the general population; (b) the preparation requires a significant amount of time by the obstetrician and health workers; (c) in emotionally disturbed or psychologically labile patients, the use of these techniques without any medication may precipitate a serious psychiatric disturbance, although this is a rare complication; (d) although the parturient may overtly show no pain, the physiologic responses and psychophysiologic mechanisms may persist, and these may prove deleterious to the mother and newborn (page 54); (e) if the technique involves marked hyperventilation, the mother may incur severe respiratory alkalosis with consequent decrease in cerebral and uterine blood flows, whereas, if the parturient practices fast, shallow panting breathing, hypoventilation with consequent respiratory acidosis will result, and these will reflect on the fetus and newborn; (f) insistence by "pursists" of these techniques that no medication be given in parturients in whom the method has not really affected the pain will result in even greater maternal deleterious emotional and physiopathologic effects. Indeed, many parturients who are psychologically prepared to consider pharmacologic analgesia as unnecssary and bad for the newborn, will experience a sense of failure and guilt in the event they are not able to go through the parturition process without drug-induced analgesia; and (g) similarly, insistence by "purists" that all patients deliver spontaneously may result in an unduly prolonged second stage. This is likely to produce maternal exhaustion and metabolic acidosis and significant neonatal depression from cord compression and/or uterine contractions.

As a result of experience and critical analysis, it is now generally agreed by members of the International Childbirth Education Association (ICEA)—composed of various types of health professionals working in the field—that in most instances the pain of parturition is not eliminated, but, rather, it is lessened, and, more importantly, anxiety is decreased and that both the parturient's ability to cope with the entire experience and her behavior are improved. Moreover, the earlier claims that childbirth can be pain free appear to be no longer essential to the public acceptance of prepared childbirth. Although some proponents of psychoprophylaxis still eschew all pharmacologic pain relief, most of them have moderated their position on this point. Today, most gravidas who decide to try this method are prepared psychologically so that they will not feel guilty or feel that they have failed if they are unable to go through the entire process without pharmacologic analgesia.

These techniques have three procedures in common: the educational, the physiotherapeutic, and the psychotherapeutic. *The educational process* is most important and effective in dispelling fear, anxiety, and apprehension due to lack of information or perhaps more often to misinformation concerning the anatomy and physiology of the reproductive process. Education can also be effective in enhancing self-concept and confidence. Moreover, additional benefits are derived from an opportunity to share experiences and concerns in a guided, group-discussion situation.

Physiotherapeutic procedures include physical exercise designed to improve the tone of the body and mind, respiratory exercise to be used during labor, and finally, relaxation. Many proponents of prepared childbirth consider breathing exercises essential to delivery of an adequate oxygen supply to the mother and fetus, to the establishment of a focus of cortical activation or distraction during contractions, and to the maintainence of relaxation. A variety of breathing patterns is advocated from deep, slow diaphragmatic to rapid, superifial sternal breaths and panting. Unfortunately, some of these patterns are conducive to either hyperventilation or hypoventilation, both of which are deleterious to the mother and the infant. Properly done, the breathing exercises are effective in distracting the parturients and, in this way, decreasing pain perception and thus have psychotherapeutic value. Similarly, the relaxation has a pain-diminishing effect and often produces hypnoid states.

The psychophysiologic or psychotherapeutic process involves the use of primary psychodynamic mechanisms that suppress fear and tension and help to control behavior and pain. These include suggestion, motivation, attention, and distraction, and other psychophysiologic processes. These all depend on the interpersonal relation between parturient and the obstetric team. In addition to the support given by the obstetrician and obstetric nurse, equally important (and at times more important) is the psychologic support that is given by the spouse and, if available, a nurse-midwife. In order for the husband to carry out this role effectively, the expectant father should attend classes with the gravida so he may be of ultimate assistance in achieving psychologic analgesia during labor. The father is also able to coach in the out-of-class practice of physiotherapeutic techniques during the pregnancy and to support, encourage, and coach the wife during the labor and delivery. In many hospitals, the father is welcome into the labor and delivery room so that he may provide constant support to his wife and share with her the excitement and joy of observing the birth of their child.

Techniques

Techniques of natural childbirth and psychoprophylaxis used currently, which can be collectively called "educated childbirth," include: (a) intensive antepartal psychologic and physiologic preparation—which includes a series of lectures and seminars, respiratory and other muscular exercises, and relaxation; (b) the specific procedures during labor—which include reinforcement of the psychologic preparation by the obstetric nurse, obstetrician, and other members of the obstetric team, and, most importantly, by the husband who will remain in

71

the labor room throughout the labor; (c) procedures intended to induce relaxation; (d) the use of small doses of pharmacologic analgesia as a supplement, if this is necessary; and (e) spontaneous delivery. The gravida is taught methods of relaxation and certain pain-reducing procedures that include: (a) the aforementioned varying patterns of breathing; (b) massage of the abdominal wall; and (c) pressure placed on the anterior superior iliac spine and certain parts of the low back which some claim to be a form of "acupressure"—a technique used by the Chinese to produce pain relief. The method of applying pressure is not only taught and explained but is also practiced during the antepartal training period.

Since the exercises and psychotherapeutic procedures vary among different groups, no attempt will be made to summarize them here. Instead, focus is placed on the educational content and suggested outline of the lectures/seminars that can be given to all parturients, whether or not they decide to use psychologic analgesia only. The content of the material that is presented depends on the goals of the program; the personality, background, and experience of the teacher; and the nature and needs of each individual plan. If the goal is to help parents to help themselves and to foster mature attitudes, basic principles are presented, and each couple is encouraged to apply those principles in order to satisfy their own requirements. Parents are encouraged to take an active part in the discussion period, to ask questions and suggest answers, to express anxieties which are often diminished when shared, and to voice common hopes and aspirations. Questions should be answered fully and frankly, but, if they prove disturbing or embarrassing to the group, private consultation is advisable. The balance between the lectures and group discussion is determined by the teacher's experience as well as by an appraisal of the individuals comprising the group. It is desirable to initiate the lectures/seminars some time in the early 2nd trimester and to give at least 6 and preferably 10 sessions spread out until the beginning of the 3rd trimester. In addition to the lectures/seminars, weekly sessions are devoted to physiotherapeutic instructions and practices. After the lecture series is completed (by the 30th–32nd week), the sessions are devoted to physical and psychologic conditioning (Table 7).

TECHNIQUES OF HYPNOSIS

Most practitioners of hypnosis for obstetric patients begin with early preparation at about the 5th or 6th month of pregnancy and subsequently thereafter every 2–4 weeks. The eye-roll method is widely used to determine the patient's susceptibility to hypnosis and selection for hypnotic analgesia. Many practitioners use phonograph records containing instructions that are played during the first session, and then the patient is asked to replay them at home. The word hypnosis is not used, but, instead, the term "medical relaxation" is substituted to suggest to the patient what is expected of her during these sessions. Many practitioners emphasize the importance of relaxation.

TABLE 7. LECTURES/SEMINARS FOR PREPARED CHILDBIRTH

First Session
  a) General orientation: purpose of the program
  b) Anatomy of the uterus: blood supply and nerve supply
  c) Anatomy of the pelvis, vagina, and external genitalia
  d) Physiology of the uterus: menstruation and conception
  e) Growth of the fetus
  f) Anatomy and function of the placenta
  g) Alterations in maternal functions during pregnancy
  h) Discussion period: questions, answers, and comments

Second Session: Physiology and Psychology of Pregnancy and Labor
  a) Physiology of uterine contraction and the auxiliary forces of labor
  b) Free discussion of unusual anxiety and apprehension
  c) False notions and misinformation
  d) Mechanisms that can be mobilized to counteract these notions
  e) Anatomic, biochemical, and physiological bases of parturition pain and factors that contribute to suffering
  f) Physical and psychologic factors that influence pain
  g) Effects of parturition pain on mother, fetus, and newborn
  h) Discussion period: questions, answers, and comments

Third Session: Obstetric Pain Relief
  a) Overview of psychological analgesia and mechanism of its action
  b) Overview of pharmacologic analgesia
  c) Benefits, advantages, disadvantages, limitations of each method
  d) Description of oxygen and anesthetic equipment
  e) Discussion: questions, answers, and comments

Fourth Session: Labor and Delivery
  a) Preparation for hospitalization
  b) Symptoms of labor
  c) Admission procedures and ongoing hospital care
  d) Husband's role during admission, labor, and delivery
  e) Maternal and fetal monitoring
  f) Possible need of episiotomy
  g) Possible need for induction of labor, forceps, or cesarean section
  h) Discussion: questions, answers, and comments
  i) Inspection of delivery room

Fifth Session: Postnatal Adjustments
  a) Immediate reactions to childbirth
  b) Care in delivery room and recovery room
  c) Physiologic and emotional changes
  d) Postpartum exercises and check-up
  e) Care of the newborn in hospital and at home, including feeding, bathing, clothing, sleep, and crying patterns.

Sixth Session
  a) Review of entire series of lectures
  b) Free discussion

Seventh Session
  a) Motion picture showing actual delivery
  b) Slides showing delivery suite

Many authorities prefer the arm levitation technique which, though somewhat time consuming, is the best means of inducing relaxation and then superimposing analgesia. For this purpose, the patient is brought into a quiet room and allowed to relax. Induction of hypnosis then begins, using the eye fixation technique. As the hypnotic state deepens, arm levitation can be induced and analgesia of the levitated arm is suggested. The patient is then instructed to transfer the analgesia from the arm to the abdomen and perineum simply by rubbing, so that relief from pain of labor and delivery can be produced. Once the patient has been appropriately trained, it is not too difficult to teach the gravida self-induction, thus making the presence of the hypnotist unnecessary.

ACUPUNCTURE ANALGESIA

Despite the great interest in China in the use of acupuncture analgesia for surgery, the use of this method in obstetrics has been limited to cesarean section and has not been used for vaginal delivery because of their cultural premise that parturition is a physiologic function and does not require analgesia. In contrast, a few western trained physicians in other parts of Asia, Europe, and North America have given acupuncture a clinical trial with conflicting results. Several reports indicate that effective analgesia was derived using electoacupuncture achieved with low frequency (2 Hz) and high intensity stimulation which elicited strong muscle contraction applied on the low back region bilaterally. The pain relief was evaluated to be good in nearly half of the women. Although the results suggested a relation between high suggestability and good analgesic effect, the pain relief was not due to suggestability alone, because both suggestion and hypnosis had been used prior to sensory stimulation without producing pain relief.

On the other hand, several obstetric anesthetists who have given acupuncture an adequate trial have not obtained satisfactory results and have discontinued its use. Since it has been shown that acupuncture stimulation, especially that entailing electroacpuncture, increases liberation of endorphins, it may be that the reason for inadequate analgesia is the lack of information of the best acupuncture points or the use of incorrect parameters for the electrical stimulation. In any case, poor results, together with the fact that electrical acupuncture may interfere with electronic monitoring of the fetus, suggests that, at present, acupuncture should have little or no role in obstetric analgesia.

TRANSCUTANEOUS ELECTRICAL NERVE STIMULATION (TENS)

This is another nonpharmacologic technique that has been given clinical trial. In one study in which two pairs of surface electrodes were taped on the parturient's back, one pair was applied on the skin overlying T_{10}-L_1 vertebrae with each electrode just lateral of the midline, while the second pair was applied bilaterally on the skin overlying $S_2 - S_4$ vertebrae. Stimulation was induced by a two-channel generator producing biphasic pulses that were variable in frequency and amplitude. A low intensity , high frequency (60–80 Hz) stimulation was applied continuously via the upper electrodes, and, as soon as more intense pain caused by the onset of uterine contractions was felt, the patient herself increased the intensity of stimulation to a level where muscular fasiculation appeared in the vicinity of the electrode and maintained this intensity for one minute. Both stimulation levels were experienced as a tingling sensation of different intensity over the involved dermatomes of the back. During both the late first stage and the second stage, high intensity stimulation was applied continuously via the sacral electrodes in addition to the thoracic stimulation. Of 147 parturients thus treated, 44% considered the relief of uterine pain to be good to very good, 44% had partial relief, while the rest had no relief. However, during the second stage, 104 had to have regional analgesia, primarily in the form of bilateral pudendal block, and 4 received epidural alangesia. No serious maternal side effects or changes in labor patterns were seen, but the sacral stimulation did interfere with the signal of the FHR monitoring. In another report, TENS gave good relief from backache to most of 50 parturients, but relief of the anterior abdominal pain was satisfactory in only 3. In view of these results, TENS may be considered as a procedure to be used in obstetric clinics where the services of an obstetrical anesthetist are not available.

MECHANISM OF ANALGESIA

The mechanism of analgesia obtained with the three psychologic techniques is unknown, but current evidence suggests that pain relief results through psychophysiologic mechanisms that inhibit transmission of nociceptive information at various levels of the neuraxis. There is ample evidence that the educational and psychotherapeutic aspects, especially when carried out in a group, are highly effective in decreasing anxiety, fear, and apprehension, and increasing motivation. The neurophysiologic evidence cited in Chapter 3 suggests that such mental activities as emotion, motivation, attention, suggestion, prior conditioning, and distraction, all of which are subserved at least in part by neocortical processes, may effect both sensory and affective aspects of pain. These mental activities, as well as those that may be generated by suggestion and the placebo effect, activate neocortical processes that, in turn, may stimulate the periaqueductal gray (PAG) neurons and thus increase the activity of this powerful descending pain-suppressing system and perhaps other descending control systems.

Studies have demonstrated that the analgesic effect of acupuncture and electrical analgesia in humans is reversible by naloxone. Moreover, acupuncture in animals has been shown to inhibit the response of dorsal horn nociceptive neurons. These results suggest that the production of partial or complete pain relief with acupuncture or electrical stimulation involves the opiate system. In contrast, naloxone had no antagnostic effect on hypnotically induced analgesia in humans. This negative result could be due to the complex nature of hypnotic analgesia which probably involves cognitive and memory factors integrated at the highest levels of the nervous system. Moreover, since it has been reported that segmental withdrawal reflexes are suppressed during hypnotic analgesia, a descending antinociceptive pathway not involving endorphins seems to be an integral component of this type of analgesia.

CHAPTER 7. SIMPLE METHODS OF OBSTETRIC ANALGESIA

In many parts of the world, the services of anesthetists or other persons trained to administer major forms of regional or general anesthesia are not available for most obstetric patients. Under such circumstances, the midwife or obstetrician must rely on the use of "simple" methods of analgesia. These usually consist of the combined use of sedatives and narcotics for most labor, and, in some instances, are followed by simple methods of inhalation analgesia or simple regional analgesia. In this chapter, the clinical use of sedatives and narcotics will be briefly described. The techniques of inhalation and regional analgesia are considered in subsequent chapters.

MANAGEMENT DURING LATENT PHASE

During the latent phase, which extends from the onset of regular uterine contractions to the time the cervix becomes 3 cm dilated, the contractions are of mild intensity and occur every 3–4 minutes. Labor pain during the latent phase is usually mild, but reaction to it varies greatly. Prepared or "educated" parturients are able to control their fears and anxieties, behave admirably, and manifest little or no discomfort. These patients usually require only moral support and reinforcement of "psychologic analgesia." Unprepared parturients, however, manifest moderate discomfort; a few complain bitterly of pain. These patients will require intensive psychologic support and sedative drugs that help to allay apprehension, anxiety, and fear.

Sedatives

Properly used, sedation to supplement psychologic support not only enhances emotional well-being, but also produces drug-induced rest and sleep. Sedation can be achieved with a variety of drugs, including ataractics or tranquilizers, short-acting barbiturates, the benzodiazepines, and a heterogeneous group of other agents.

Tranquilizers relieve apprehension and anxiety, produce tranquility and ataraxia, and reduce nausea and vomiting. During the latent phase, promazine (Sparine), hydroxyzine (Vistaril), and promethazine (Phenergan) given in doses of 50 mg intramuscularly or in increments of 15–25 mg intravenously are highly effective sedatives and reduce anxiety. Possible side effects of some phenothiazine derivatives such as chlorpromazine (Thorazine) and perphenazine (Trilafon) include orthostatic hypotension and extrapryamidal motor disturbances. Some clinicians combine one of these drugs with 50–75 mg of meperidine during the latent phase, but, for reasons given below, it is important not to administer narcotics until labor has progressed into the active phase. The claim that these drugs potentiate the actions of analagesics and anesthetics has not been borne out by controlled clinical trials. In fact, experimental studies indicate that some of these agents have anti-analgesic action. In any case, the combination should be avoided, certainly during the latent phase.

Short-acting barbiturates such as pentobarbital (Nembutal) and secobarbital (Seconal) are still widely used by some obstetricians, especially as hypnotics and as sedatives. For these purposes, the average parturient will require 100 mg of one of these agents by mouth. However, in many hospitals, barbiturates are no longer used to induce sleep because of the prolonged retention time of barbiturates in both maternal and fetal tissues and the hangover experienced by many patients.

Diazepam (Valium) has become widely used in many obstetric centers in North America and Europe. Intramuscular doses of 10 mg or intravenous injection of 5 mg of diazepam produce amnesia and reduce maternal anxiety and apprehension. In addition to its efficacy as a sedative, diazepam has been found to raise the threshold to the systemic toxicity of local anesthetics and therefore its use may be indicated prior to the use of regional anesthesia. However, as previously mentioned, diazepam used in amounts of doses larger than 10 mg intramuscularly or smaller doses given rapidly intravenously has been known to produce the following effects in the newborn: hypotonia, decreased sucking, hypothermia, hyperactivity, and some respiratory depression. These undesirable side effects may be even more pronounced in the preterm or otherwise compromised infant.

Scopolamine has been used widely in obstetrics for over 70 years. In optimum doses (0.3–0.6 mg) it produces no analgesia but does produce mild sedation and tranquility, with some amnesia and usually intense dryness of the mouth. Many patients consider the dryness very uncomfortable, and it may be the primary reason for the restlessness seen following the use of this agent. Since, currently, there are better sedatives and tranquilizers and since many parturients prefer to remember their labor, there is no justification for its routine use in obstetrics.

ANALGESICS DURING THE ACTIVE PHASE OF LABOR

The active phase of labor begins when the cervix is dilated 3 cm or more and ends when complete cervical dilation occurs. The active phase usually lasts 4–5 hours in primigravidas and about 2 hours in multiparas. During this phase, uterine contractions progressively increase in intensity from about 25 or 30 mm Hg to about 50 mm Hg, the duration increases from about 40 to 60 seconds or more, and their frequency from 2–3 to 4–5 contractions per 10 minutes. There is a commensurate increase in the intensity of pain from mild to moderate at the beginning of the period, to maximum intensty when the cervix becomes fully dilated.

Patients who have been prepared for natural childbirth or psychoprophylaxis are usually able to get along well until the latter part of the active phase when uterine contractions become so severe that psychologic analgesia needs to be reinforced with drug-induced analgesia. The parturient who has had psychologic preparation during pregnancy, but who does not plan to deliver without help of drug-induced analgesia, will require some medication throughout the active phase. At the other end of the spectrum, is the parturient who has not had the benefit of such preparation and who will require significant drug-induced analgesia. A combination of a sedative and narcotic or narcotic combined with inhalation analgesia or paracervical block is usually sufficient until the last part of the active phase and may even prove adequate until the actual delivery.

Narcotic Analgesics

Narcotics are the most widely used drugs given to parturients to relieve the pain of childbirth. However, their use should be reserved for the active phase of labor, because, given prematurely, narcotics significantly prolong the latent phase, probably by interfering with the very complex interrelated factors responsible for the "acceleration phase." This is the interval of labor that is the transition from the slow rate of progress, characteristic of the latent phase, to the rapid progress, characteristic of the phase of maximum slope. The only exceptions to this rule of strictly avoiding narcotics during the latent and acceleration phases are: the unusual parturient who experiences severe pain during this period; the uninformed, unprepared primigravida (especially a teenager) who is extremely anxious and apprehensive; and the parturient with very slow progress and unusually prolonged labor. In many of these patients, fear and anxiety cause or aggravate incoordinate uterine contractions which are primarily responsible for the slow progress. In such patients, the administration of a narcotic, especially morphine, proves very beneficial. Finally, a narcotic in combination with a sedative maybe indicated in primigravidas whose onset of labor occurs in the evening and it is deemed advisable to assure her a good night's sleep free from discomfort so that she is well rested when the active phase begins.

It is generally known that narcotics effect analgesia, pleasant modification of mood, relief from anxiety and fear, physical and mental relaxation, and, if the parturient is tired, sleep between contractions. These, together with the fact that they are inexpensive and simple to administer, are responsible for their widespread popularity. On the other hand, narcotics rarely completely relieve severe pain. Rather, they provide adequate (satisfactory) relief to about 70–80% of those with moderate pain and to about 25% of those with severe pain, with the rest deriving only inadequate analgesia. Moreover, these drugs produce undesirable side effects in the mother. They are specific depressants of neonatal respiration and central nervous system and invariably produce a depressed ENNS score. Moreover, when used prematurely or in excessive doses, they slow up labor except in patients in whom labor is being stimulated with oxytocin. Narcotics are contraindicated in parturients who have been receiving a monoamine oxidase inhibitor before labor, since they may sustain a long period of marked hypotension and coma. Numerous well controlled clinical trials (mostly in surgical patients) suggest that, in equipotent doses, narcotics produce similar degrees of analgesia and side effects but the duration of relief varies with each drug. However, there is some indirect evidence to show that meperidine (Demerol, Pethidine) passes the blood brain barrier of newborn infants with greater difficulty and, consequently, there is theoretically less neonatal depression than after morphine.

To obtain optimal results with narcotics (maximum analgesia with little or no side effects), it is essential to administer these agents in optimal doses via the optimal route and at the appropriate time. For patients with moderate pain, which is usually experienced at the beginning of the phase of maximum slope and after the cervix is 4 cm dilated, it is best to give these drugs intramuscularly, usually in doses of from 75–100 mg of meperidine (Demerol, Pethidine) or equipotent doses of other narcotics. Adequate analgesia will occur in 15–20 minutes and will last 2–4 hours, depending on the drug. Several well controlled studies have shown that following intramuscular administration, the incidence of neonatal depression is highest when the delivery occurs about 3 hours after injection and is lowest when it occurs within 1 hour or after 4 hours after the injection. In parturients who have severe pain of the late active phase and for those who are progressing rapidly, it is best to give these agents intravenously slowly. Doses of 25–40 mg of meperidine or equipotent doses of other drugs provide ample analgesia within about 5 minutes and this lasts for about 1½–2 hours.

Premixed Solutions of Narcotics and Narcotic Antagonists. These have been advocated and used by some clinicians, particularly in Great Britain, because they are said to produce analgesia without concomitant depression of the mother and newborn. Unfortunately, these claims have not been borne out by careful clnical trials, some of which have actually shown that these premixed solutions produced less analgesia, more side effects, and did not reduce the incidence of neonatal depression. For these reasons, premixed solutions have been abandoned in many quarters and are not recommended for routine use in obstetrics. On the other hand, if neonatal depression is considered to be due to narcotics, a narcotic antagonist may be given to the newborn. Of the several currently available, naloxone (Narcan) is by far the best because it is a specific narcotic antagonist without possessing the propensity of neonatal respiratory depression or other side effects of its own, as is characteristic with the others. The recommended dose for reversal of neonatal narcotic depression is 5μg/kg given intramuscularly.

SUPPLEMENTAL ANALGESIA

When sedatives and narcotics are no longer effective in relieving severe pain, additional pain relief can be afforded the parturient by administering inhalation analgesia or a paracervical block. After the onset of the second stage, when perineal pain becomes progressively more severe, bilateral pudendal block is probably the best simple method of relieving it. If for some reason this procedure cannot be done, infiltration of the perineum with very dilute solutions of local anesthetic can be used as a substitute. Infiltration is particularly useful for the incision and repair of episiotomy.

CHAPTER 8. REGIONAL ANALGESIA-ANESTHESIA FOR LABOR AND VAGINAL DELIVERY

GENERAL CONSIDERATIONS

In the past three decades there has been an impressive and progressive increase in the use of regional analgesia-anesthesia during labor and for delivery, not only in the United States but in many other countries where heretofore pharmacologic obstetric anesthesia has been avoided. The most common techniques are: (1) continuous epidural block; (2) subarachnoid (saddle) block; (3) bilateral paracervical and/or bilateral pudendal block; and (4) continuous caudal block (Figure 36).

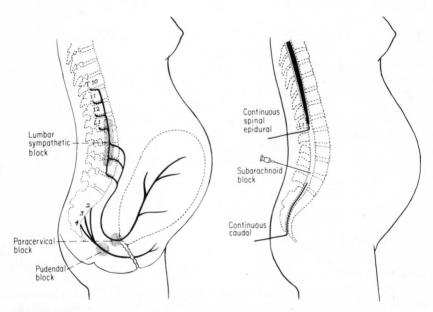

FIGURE 36. Regional anesthetic techniques used for obstetric analgesia-anesthesia. Lumbar sympathetic block is rarely used but is highly effective in relieving pain of the first stage and may be preferable to paracervical block, especially in high risk pregnancies. (Modified from and courtesy of Bonica, J.J.: An atlas on mechanisms and pathways of pain in labor. What's New, 217:16, 1960.)

The reason for the widespread popularity of regional analgesia is that when each technique is properly applied it affords the following significant advantages: (1) in contrast to narcotics, regional analgesia produces complete relief of pain in most parturients; (2) the hazard of pulmonary aspiration of gastric contents during general anesthesia is virtually eliminated; (3) provided it is properly administered and no complications occur, regional anesthesia causes no maternal or neonatal depression; (4) administered at the proper time, it does not impede the progress of labor; (5) continuous techniques can be extended for the delivery and may even be modified for cesarean section if this becomes necessary; (6) regional analgesia permits the mother to remain awake during labor and delivery so that she can experience the pleasure of actively participating in the birth of her child; and (7) provided the mother is doing well, the anesthetist can leave her and resuscitate the newborn if this is necessary.

The disadvantages of regional anesthesia are: (1) it requires greater skill to administer than do systemic drugs or inhalation agents; (2) technical failures occur, even in experienced hands; (3) certain techniques produce side effects that, if not properly treated, can progress to complication; (4) techniques that produce perineal muscle paralysis interfere with the mechanism of internal rotation and increase the incidence of persistent posterior positions; and (5) these procedures can only be carried out in the hospital. The contraindications to regional anesthesia are summarized on Table 8.

TABLE 8.   ABSOLUTE CONTRAINDICATIONS TO REGIONAL ANESTHESIA

1. Lack of skill and experience by administrator in technique in management of patients and in therapy of complications
2. Infection of puncture site
3. Coagulation defects   } especially for subarachnoid and extradural blocks
4. Hemorrhagic hypovolemia or shock
5. Patient's refusal or intense fear of regional anesthesia
6. Lack of experience or appreciation by obstetrician of how procedure influences management of labor

REQUISITES FOR OPTIMAL RESULTS

In order to achieve the stated objectives of obstetric analgesia, i.e., good maternal pain relief with little or no risk to her or her infant, it is essential for the physician to fulfill certain requisites:

1. He or she must know well the pain pathways of labor, the pharmacology of local anesthetics, and must have acquired sufficient skill and experience with the techniques and know how to manage the patient after regional analgesia has been administered.

2. He or she must know the possible complications, their prevention, and prompt treatment.

3. *None of the regional procedures should be begun without an intravenous infusion running and without having—for immediate use—equipment for treatment of complications and for resuscitation.*

4. Each regional technique has contraindications that must be observed.

5. Except in circumstances in which the use of a regional technique is especially indicated and provides significant advantages over all other methods, it should not be used against the wishes of the parturient.

6. Regional analgesics should not be started until the cervix is dilated 3–4 cm in multiparas and 5–6 cm in primiparas, the contractions are strong, last 35–40 seconds or more, and occur at intervals of 3 minutes or less. The only exceptions to this rule are with patients who experience extreme pain during the latent phase of labor, or with patients in whom labor has been induced and maintained with oxytocin.

7. During and following administration of the analgesia, the parturient should be given attention continuously and must be carefully observed and her blood pressure, pulse, and respiration measured every ½ minute during the first 15 minutes and every 5 minutes thereafter.

8. Frequently, it is necessary to complement these procedures with psychologic support and a sedative and, occasionally, a narcotic.

9. Personnel must be skilled and willing to supervise the patient properly.

10. Contraindications to regional anesthesia must be rigidly observed. (See Table 8.)

PHARMACOLOGY OF LOCAL ANESTHETICS

Mechanism of Action

Local anesthetic solutions are salts, usually hydrochlorides, that combine a weak base with a strong acid. In solution, the salts of local anesthetic compounds exist both in the form of uncharged (free) base (B) and as positively charged cations (BH^+). The relative proportion between the uncharged base and the charged cations depends on the pH of the solution and on the pKa of the specific drug. Since the pKa is constant for any agent, the relative proportion of free base and charged cation in the local anesthetic solution depends essentially on the pH of the solution ($BH^+ \leqq B + H^+$). When injected into the body, the slightly alkaline extracellular fluids cause the equilibrium to be shifted toward the free-base form, and relatively more of the drug will exist in the free base than as the charged cation.

Both the uncharged base form and the charged cationic form of the local anesthetic drug are involved in the total process of penetration and block of nerve conduction. The uncharged or undissociated base form is responsible for the diffusion of the drug through the nerve sheath. After penetration of the sheath, re-equilibrium occurs between the base and cationic form, and, at the cell membrane itself, the charged cations displace calcium from lipoprotein receptive sites located on the internal surface of the cell membrane and binds to them. The binding of the local anesthetic moiety to the receptive site results in blockade of the membrane's sodium channel, which, in turn, decreases sodium permeability and inhibits membrane depolarization. The mechanism of this anesthetic action is summarized in Figure 37.

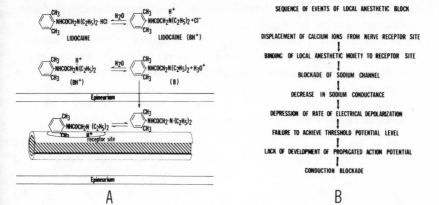

A   B

FIGURE 37. Mechanism of action of local anesthetics. The figure on the left summarizes the diffusion of base form of the local anesthetic agent across epineurium and subsequent binding of cationic form with receptor site of nerve membrane. On the right, the sequence of events of local anesthetic block. After the agent penetrates the sheath and the charged cation displaces calcium ions from the nerve receptor site, it binds to it. (See text for details.) (Courtesy of Covino, B.J., and Vassallo, H.: *Local Anesthetics. Mechanisms of Action and Clinical Use*, New York, Grune and Stratton, Inc. 1976.)

Pharmacokinetics

With infiltration techniques, the anesthetic reaches nerve endings quickly so the onset of anesthesia is very rapid. With field block and major nerve blocks, the anesthetic must reach the core of each nerve. To do this, it must penetrate the epineurium, perineurium, endoneurium, fat, blood vessels, and lymphatics that make up as much as 40% of the diameter of nerve trunks. Consequently, the onset of anesthesia takes minutes and varies directly with the nerve's diameter.

The degree of anesthesia depends upon the potency of the drug and the amount that reaches the target (nerve fibers). This, in turn, depends upon the amount of drug injected, its characteristics, and the rate of absorption into the circulation. The greater the amount absorbed, the less that is available to block nerves. The rate of absorption also influences the toxicity of local anesthetics. (See below.)

Absorption (uptake) depends on the vascularity of the injection site and the drug's solubility in tissues at the site, its breakdown rate, its concentration, and its penetration. Since local anesthetics (except cocaine) cause local vasomotor paralysis and thus increase local blood flow, this action enhances absorption. The higher the concentration of the drug, the greater the local vasomotor action. Decreased vascularity caused by hypotension or simultaneous injection of a vasoconstrictor retards absorption.

Distribution of the local anesthetic depends on regional blood flow and pH and the drug's penetrance, fat and water solubility, and the protein-binding rate. The more penetrant the local anesthetic, the more readily it will pass fibrous barriers and the more drug will reach nerve elements. The greater the fat solubility of the drug, the more drug is distributed to fat tissue (including nerves). Since local anesthetics diffuse from tissues of high pH to those of low pH, acidosis enhances absorption into the blood. Protein binding and uptake by blood plasma and erythrocytes significantly influence the distribution of local anesthetics. The most important physical characteristics that influence pharmacokinetics and anesthetic action are listed in Table 9.

Placental Transfer. All of these factors also influence the placental transfer of these agents. Since the nonionized (undissociated) moiety enhances placental transfer and since those local anesthetics with pKa closer to physiologic pH (such as mepivacaine and bupivacaine) have greater amounts of nonionized than ionized moieties, they transfer more readily. Once the drug enters the fetal blood with pH lower than the pH of maternal blood, there is a shift to the left, and if fetal acidosis occurs, ionized drug remains trapped on the fetal side of the placenta. Because the nonionized moiety continues to equilibrate on both sides of the placental membrane, a high concentration of local anesthetic develops in the fetus. In pregnant ewes, a pH gradient of 0.5 between mother and fetus results in a signifcant increase in fetal bupivacaine concentration and UV/M bupivacaine ratio.

Because only free base can traverse the placenta, maternal protein binding limits the amount of drug transfer. Consequently, less amounts of local anesthetics that are highly bound are transferred than those with lower binding capacities such as lidocaine and mepivacaine. Moreover, since protein binding capacity is concentration dependent, proportionately more drug is bound at lower maternal concentrations than obtains in higher concentrations. Another important factor that influences placental transfer is the uptake of local anesthetic by fetal tissue. Although the UV/M ratio for etidocaine is lowest in comparison with others, the uptake of this drug by fetal tissue is much greater than that of lidocaine and, consequently, the same proportion of injected lidocaine and etidocaine can be recovered from the fetus. Delivery of drug and subsequent transfer across the placenta are decreased by diminished diffusion of fetal placental units secondary to maternal hypotension.

Biotransformation

The ester type local anesthetics (procaine, chloroprocaine, and tetracaine) are hydrolyzed by pseudocholinesterase (plasma cholinesterase) in plasma while the amide drugs (lidocaine, mepivacaine, prilocaine, bupivacaine, and etidocaine) are metabolized by the microsomal enzymes of the liver. Because of its rapid hydrolysis by plasma cholinesterase, the systemic toxicity of 2-chloroprocaine, both for the mother and the fetus, is the lowest. From the point of view of the possible systemic toxicity of these agents in the newborn, it should be re-

TABLE 9. PHYSICOCHEMICAL CHARACTERISTICS OF LOCAL ANESTHETICS

	PRO-CAINE (Novo-caine)	2-CHLORO-PROCAINE (Nesa-caine)	LIDO-CAINE (Xylo-caine)	MEPIVA-CAINE (Carbo-caine)	PRILO-CAINE (Cita-nest)	TETRA-CAINE (Ponto-caine)	BUPIVA-CAINE (Mar-caine)	ETIDO-CAINE (Dura-nest)
Molecular Weight (Base)	236	307	234	246	257	264	288	276
Potency* Ratio	1	2	3	3	3	15	15	15
Toxicity* Ratio	1	0.5	2	2.5	1.5	10	10	10
Anesthetic Index	1	2	1.5	1.25	2	1.5	1.5	1.5
pKa	8.9	8.7	7.9	7.6	–	8.2	8.1	7.7
Protein Binding Maternal	66	–	64	77	55	75	95	94
Fetal	–	–	25	–	–	–	65	–
Percent Nonionized at pH 7.4	3	4.8	7.4	39	–	14	17	33
Partition Coefficient (n-Heptane 7.4)	0.6	–	2.9	0.8	0.4	–	27.5	141
Maternal Arterial Concentration	–	–	1.2–3.5	2.0–7.0	1.0–1.5	–	0.26	0.25–1.3
Umbilical Vein Concentration	–	–	0.8–1.8	2.0–5.0	1.1–1.5	–	0.08–0.1	>0.07–0.45
UV/M Ratio	–	–	0.5–0.7	0.7–0.72	1.0–1.2	–	0.3–0.44	0.14–0.35
Half-Life Adult	–	21 sec	1.6 hr	1.9 hr	–	–	9.4 hr	2.6 hr
Newborn	–	43 sec	3.0 hr	9.0 hr	–	–	8.1 hr	–

* Procaine used as standard of reference = 1. Ratios vary according to technique of regional anesthesia used.

membered that: (a) the microsomal enzymes of the liver responsible for their metabolic breakdown are not fully developed in the newborn; (b) renal excretion of the unchanged molecule is slower in the newborn than in older infants or adults; and (c) the permeability of the blood-brain barrier is greater in the newborn than later in life.

Clinical Characteristics

To select the optimal local anesthetic drug for a particular regional anesthetic procedure in a particular parturient and under specific circumstances, it is necessary to consider the characteristics of those drugs indicated in Table 10. In addition to the aforementioned factors (protein binding, UV/M ratios, pKa, and percent of nonionized drug at pH 7.4), it is also necessary to consider: (a) anesthetic activity or potency; (b) latency or induction time; (c) penetrance; (d) duration of action; and (e) local and general toxicity.

TABLE 10. CLINICAL CHARACTERISTICS AND CONCENTRATIONS OF LOCAL ANESTHETICS

		PRO-CAINE (Novocaine)	2-CHLORO-PROCAINE (Nesacaine)	LIDO-CAINE (Xylocaine)	MEPIVA-CAINE (Carbocaine)	PRILO-CAINE (Citanest)	TETRA-CAINE (Pontocaine)	BUPIVA-CAINE (Marcaine)	ETIDO-CAINE (Duranest)
CHARACTERISTICS	Anesthetic Potency Ratio	1	2	3	3	3	15	15	15
	Latency	Moderate	Fast	Fast	Moderate	Moderate	Very Slow	Fast	Very Fast
	Penetrance	Moderate	Marked	Marked	Moderate	Moderate	Poor	Moderate	Moderate
	Duration	Short	Very Short	Moderate	Moderate	Moderate	Long	Long	Long
	(Ratio)	1	0.75	2	2	1.75	6–8	6–8	6–8
CONCENTRATIONS (%)	Infiltration	0.5	0.5	0.25	0.25	0.25	0.05	0.05	0.1
	Field Block	0.75	0.75	0.5	0.5	0.5	0.1	0.1	0.2
	Pudendal/Paracervical	1.5	1.5	0.75–1.0	0.75–1.0	0.75–1.0	0.15	0.125	0.37
	Extradural Block Analgesia	1.5	1.5	0.5–1.0	0.5–1.0	0.5–1.0	0.2	0.125–0.25	0.5–0.75
	Motor Block	3	3	2	2	2	0.4	0.5–0.75	1.0–1.5
	Maximum Amount (mg/kg)	12	15	6	6	6	2	2	2

The absolute potency and absolute toxicity of local anesthetic drugs described by pharmacologists is of little importance to the clinician. He should be concerned primarily with relative toxicity and therapeutic (anesthetic) index. For example, milligram per milligram, tetracaine (Pontocaine) is 10 times as toxic as procaine (relative toxicity ratio, 10), but, since tetracaine is so potent, it produces the same degree of anesthesia in 1/15 the dose of procaine (relative potency ratio 15). Its corrected toxicity ratio is 0.66 and its anesthetic index is 1.5. In other words, in equianesthetic concentrations, tetracaine is actually less toxic than procaine and has the advantage of producing analgesia that lasts approximately 3 times as long as that produced by procaine.

Latency or time required for onset of anesthesia is one of the properties of local anesthetics important to the clinician. This depends on: (1) anesthetic activity;

(2) concentration and total dose; (3) distance from the site of action; and (4) penetrance of the compound. The *penetrance* (its inherent ability to penetrate fibrous tissue and other structures between the site of injection and the individual nerve fibers) is another clinically important property of the local anesthetics: the more penetrant the agent, the quicker and more intense the anesthesia. The *duration* of anesthesia depends primarily on the activity of the drug, its concentration, the total dose, and the vascularity of the region.

Table 10 summarizes the clinical characteristics and optimal concentrations of local anesthetics currently available. Although procaine was used most widely during the 50 years after it was introduced in clinical practice and even today is considered the standard of reference, it is used infrequently for obstetric analgesia, primarily because of its short duration of action and intermediate latency and penetrance. Similarly, although tetracaine (Pontocaine) produces prolonged analgesia, it is rarely used for regional analgesia other than subarachnoid block because of its very prolonged (slow) latency and poor penetrance. Initially, prilocaine (Citanest) was considered the ideal local anesthetic for obstetric patients, but clinical usefullness was curtailed by the high incidence of methemoglobinemia. Until the advent of bupivacaine, lidocaine and mepivacaine were the most widely used local anesthetics in obstetric practice, but the findings that both agents used to achieve epidural analgesia caused low ENNS scores, especially a significant decrease in muscle strength and tone, have cause most obstetric anesthesiologists and obstetricians to discontinue their use in obstetric analgesia. The most recent addition, etidocaine (Duranest), has the obvious advantage of high protein binding, short latency, high penetrance, and long duration, but, because it produces profound motor block, it is not used to achieve analgesia for vaginal delivery, although it is the ideal drug to produce perineal relaxation after internal rotation of the descending part. (See page 112.)

As a result of the aforementioned consideration, until recently, 2-chloroprocaine (Nesacaine) and bupivacaine (Marcaine) have been the most frequently used agents for obstetric analgesia. Because of its low systemic toxicity, 2-chloroprocaine has been the agent of choice in high-risk pregnancies (e.g., toxemia, eclampsia, prematurity). However, the published reports of a number of cases of very prolonged neural blockade and, in some instances, persistent neurologic deficit and symptomatology of adhesive arachnoiditis following the accidental subarachnoid administration of 2-chloroprocaine intended for epidural analgesia have caused a signifcant number of obstetric departments to discontinue the use of this otherwise very valuable drug for epidural block. Nevertheless, 2-chloroprocaine is still the local anesthetic drug of choice to achieve local infiltration, field block, and paracervical/pudendal blocks.

Addition of Epinephrine. In the first edition of this brochure, the addition of epinephrine to the local anesthetic agent was advocated for several reasons. Epinephrine produces local vasoconstriction and thus decreases regional blood flow and retards the drug's absorption by the blood, resulting in more drug left in the target (nerve area). Consequently, the latency or induction time is shortened, the intensity and duration of analgesia is increased, and the risk of systemic toxicity is reduced. Moreover, epinephrine counteracts depressant effects of large local anesthetic doses on the myocardium and vascular system. While this is still true, the more frequent use of small volumes and low concentrations of bupivacaine make the addition of epinephrine no longer essential. This, together with the fact that amounts of 25–30 μg of epinephrine may decrease myometrial contractility, has caused many anesthetists to discontinue the use of vasoconstrictors. It deserves emphasis, however, that epinephrine should be added to the local anesthetic solution if large volumes and high concentrations of bupivacaine are used for epidural anesthesia for cesarean section or high concentrations of lidocaine or mepivacaine are used for vaginal delivery.

In the event that it is desirable to have the vasoconstrictor in the local anesthetic solution, add the epinephrine just before the administration rather than use solutions that contain epinephrine added by the manufacturer. Although this adds an extra step to the procedure, there are important reasons why this should be done. Since local anesthetic solutions containing epinephrine have a pH ranging from 3.78–4.06, they require much more buffering by body fluids in order to hydrolyze the anesthetic and free the base. This increases the induction time and may decrease the intensity and duration of the regional anesthetic. Moreover, solutions with such low pH often cause significant local irritation, and, if the solution is accidentally injected into the subarachnoid space, it may cause severe vasoconstriction leading to a "spinal artery blood syndrome." Indeed, a group of consultants who were asked to review and discuss the possible etiology of the prolonged sensory and motor deficits and neurologic sequelae that have followed the accidental injection of large volumes of chloroprocaine into the subarachnoid space suggested that the low pH of this drug (3.167 for a 2% solution and 3.126 for the 3% solution) may have caused acidification of the cerebrospinal fluid, which is known to have poor buffering capacity. This problem can be obviated by adding fresh epinephrine to the plain solution of bupivacaine (which has a pH of 4.975 for the 1% solution) or lidocaine (which has a pH of 6.137 for the 1% solution). The optimal concentration of epinephrine is 1:200,-000, or 5 mg/ml. The only way to measure the epinephrine accurately is to use a 0.25 ml tuberculin syringe and add a 0.1 ml of 1:1,000 epinephrine solution to each 20 ml of local anesthetic solution.*

---

*1 ml of 1:1,000 solution contains 1 mg (or 1,000 μg) of epinephrine. Therefore, 0.1 ml contans 0.1 mg or 100 μg; added to 20 ml it results in 5 μg/ml.

COMPLICATIONS OF REGIONAL ANESTHESIA

Virtually all regional anesthetic techniques administered to parturients have consistent side effects that, unless properly managed, can progress to complications. (There is a great difference between side effects and complications) Side effects include: (a) vasomotor blockade inherent in subarachnoid, spinal epidural, and caudal blocks (and to a lesser extent, the rarely used lumbar sympathetic block) that if not properly managed can produce arterial hypotension; (b) absorption of the local anesthetic drug into the circulation which, if excessive, will produce systemic toxic reactions; (c) placental transfer of the local anesthetic which may be sufficient to produce fetal depression. In addition, improper technique in inducing epidural or caudal analgesia can result in dural puncture, and, unless this is diagnosed prior to injection, total spinal anesthetia will develop. Puncture of the dura inherent in subarachnoid block or produced accidentally during induction of extradural block may produce postpuncture headache. Finally, improper technique can lead to very rare neurological complications. To avoid repetition in subsequent chapters, these side effects and complications will be discussed here under the following headings: (a) maternal hypotension; (b) systemic toxic reactions; (c) fetal depression from local anesthetics; (d) Postpuncture headache; (e) high or total spinal anesthesia; (f) urinary retention; and (g) neurologic complications.

Maternal Hypotension

Although vasomotor block is inherent in subarachnoid, spinal epidural, and caudal anesthesia, the degree of consequent hypotension is usually minimal, provided that the patient is well hydrated, lies on her side after induction of the block, and the level of analgesia does not extend above T_{10}. If severe hypotension does develop, it is most likely caused by concommitant compression of the aorta and vena cava by the gravid uterus. Hypotension associated with extradural analgesia develops less precipitously and is of lesser intensity than with subarachnoid block, probably because the slow onset of block permits the parturient to better mobilize compensatory mechanisms.

The effects of maternal hypotension on the mother, progress of labor, and the fetus and newborn depend on: (a) the severity and duration of hypotension; (b) the type and stage of labor; and (c) whether or not complications are present. With transient, mild, or moderate hypotension, the normovolemic parturient and her fetus sustain no serious effects, and uterine contractions are unaffected. On the other hand, persistent moderate hypotension or severe hypotension, even of brief duration, may have serious side effects on the mother and decrease uteroplacental blood flow, with consequent diminution of the transfer of blood gases and nutrients across the placenta. The harmful effects of persistent maternal hypotension are manifested by serious fetal bradycardia (late decelerations) and acidosis and by neonatal depression and metabolic acidosis.

The incidence and magnitude of hypotension can be significantly decreased by: (a) not using these methods in patients with hypovolemia or those with severe supine hypotensive syndrome; (b) giving a prophylactic infusion of 800–1,000 ml of lactated Ringer's solution within the 20 minutes just prior to induction of analgesia; (c) properly carrying out the procedure so that the level of analgesia does not extend above the tenth thoracic dermatome; (d) having the parturient be on her side after the block is established; and (e) measuring the blood pressure every 30 seconds for the first 15 minutes after the block is instituted in order to detect promptly the onset of hypotension. If hypotension begins to develop, the parturient should be asked to change sides. In the event she is in the lithotomy position ready to deliver, lateral uterine displacement (LUD) is effected manually, with the Colon-Morales or Kennedy displacer, or by having the parturient tilted to the left and placing a wedge under her right buttock. If these maneuvers prove ineffective, ephedrine is given intravenously in increments of 5–10 mg. Methoxamine (Vasoxyl), phenylephrine (Neosynephrine), and metaraminol (Aramine) should *not* be given because they produce uterine vasoconstriction with further decrease of intervillous perfusion and fetal bradycardia (Figure 38).

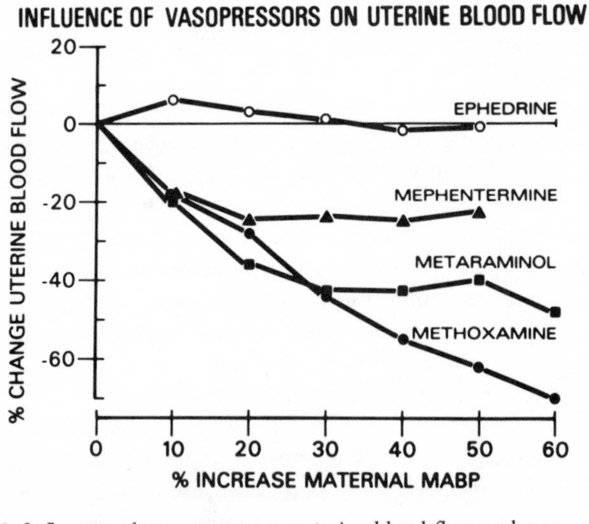

INFLUENCE OF VASOPRESSORS ON UTERINE BLOOD FLOW

FIGURE 38. Influence of vasopressors on uterine blood flow and mean arterial pressure (MABP). Note that ephedrine does not influence uterine blood flow even with doses that increase maternal MABP as much as 50%. On the other hand, other vasopressors decrease uterine blood flow, and the greater the increase in MABP (and presumably the greater the dose of the vasopressor) the greater the decrease in uterine blood flow. (Courtesy of Bromage, P.R.: *Epidural Anagesia*, Philadelphia, W.B. Saunders Co., 1978; developed from data by Ralston, D., Shnider, S., and deLorimier, A.: Anesthesiology 40:354, 1974.)

Systemic Toxic Reactions

Systemic toxic reactions occur when the local anesthetic is administered in such fasion that the rate of absorption greatly exceeds the rate of biotransformation and elimination by the body. This may be due to (1) injection of an excessive dose; (2) accidental intravascular injection of a therapeutic dose; (3) the rate of absorption being much faster than normal; and (4) the rate of detoxification being abnormally slow. As a result, the amount of the local anesthetic in the circulation increases to a toxic threshold level. In obstetric patients, the first two listed above are the most important causes.

Symptomatology. Toxic reactions may be arbitrarily classified as *mild, moderate,* and *severe. Mild reactions* occur when the blood level in the circulation is just above physiologic limits and are manifested by palpitation, a metallic taste, dryness of the mouth and throat, tinnitus, vertigo, dysarthria, apprehension and nausea, excitement and confusion. *Moderate reactions* are manifested by severe confusion and muscular twitchings that progress to convulsions. *Severe reactions* result from massive overdosage of the drug and are manifested by severe hypotension, bradycardia, and respiratory depression which may progress to cardiovascular standstill and respiratory arrest.

The fetus and newborn are invariably depressed as a result of matenal asphyxia or severe hypertension or uterine tetanic contractions that occassionally develop during convulsions. Each of these factors impairs placental gas transfer and produces fetal hypoxia, hypercarbia, and acidosis, all of which markedly depress the cardiovascular and central nervous systems of the newborn. These latter effects may be aggravated by the placental transfer of large amounts of the local anesthetic.

These serious complications can and must be avoided by: using the smallest concentration and volume of local anesthetic that assures good results; use of epinephrine 1:200,000 to retard the rate of absorption if unusually large volumes and concentrations of local anesthetics are used for epidural block for cesarean section (e.g., 20 ml of 2% lidocaine or mepivacaine); and, most important, making sure that the point of the needle or catheter is not in a blood vessel before each injection.

Treatment. Mild reactions are treated by close observation and encouragement of the patient and administration of oxygen. Convulsions must be treated *immediately* so that the mother and fetus do not suffer asphyxia. Oxygen is administered promptly under positive pressure and muscular activity is controlled by the intravenous injection of 60–100 mg of succinylcholine. In addition, 5–10 mg of diazepam or 50–100 mg of thiopental should be given to control seizure activity of the cerebral cortex. If any difficulty is encountered in keeping the airway patent, tracheal intubation is promptly carried out. Care must be taken to avoid administering a large dose of barbiturates which in itself produces myocardial depression. Repeated small doses may be administered if required. Severe reactions require support of the circulation with fluids and vasopressors as well as artificial ventilation. As already mentioned, systemic absorption reactions are least likely to occur with 2-chloroprocaine (Nesacaine) except after inadvertent intravascular administration of a large dose. Even under those circumstances, the reaction is short-lasting, usually less than 6 minutes.

Fetal Depression From Local Anesthetics

In addition the the mechanisms mentioned in the preceeding section, high fetal blood levels of local anesthetics can occur: (1) from accidental injection of the drug into the fetus during attempts at caudal block or paracervical block; (2) accidental injection into the uterine artery during attempts at paracervical block; and (3) injection into the myometrium or rapid diffusion across the uterine arterial wall so that much of the drug is diverted directly to the intervillous space, across the placental membrane, and into the fetus. In all of these instances, the fetal blood levels will be significantly higher than the maternal. To minimize the incidence of this complication of paracervical block it is essential to: (a) use the smallest concentration and volume that will produce good results to keep the total dose as low as possible; and (b) use careful technique avoiding accidental intraarterial injection.

Postpuncture Headache

A diagnosis of postpuncture (postspinal) headache is made if a known or suspected dural puncture has occurred and the headache is precipitated or aggravated by elevation of the head or sitting or standing and is virtually and promptly eliminated when the puerpera lies down. The headache is usually located in the forehead just behind the eyes and occasionally radiates to both temples and to the occipital and suboccipital regions. It may be mild, moderate, or severe. It is caused by the loss of cerebrospinal fluid through the hole in the dura created by the needle puncture. When the patient sits or stands, the lowered cerebrospinal fluid pressure permits displacement of the brain and brainstem caudad, resulting in traction on blood vessels and other pain sensitive structures in the cranium. The amount of fluid lost depends primarily on the size of the hole in the dura, the position of the parturient during and after the puncture, and the hydration level of the puerpera. The relation of the needle size and incidence of headache is as follows: 25–35% with 18 gauge; 10–20% with 20 gauge; 8–15% with 22 gauge; 2–5% with 24 gauge; less than 3% with 25 or 26 gauge. In the puerpera, the incidence of headache is greater than in nonpregnant patients because of: (a) withholding of fluids, diaphoresis, and blood loss during delivery; (b) bearing-down efforts during the second stage increase CSF loss; (c) diuresis in the postpartum period produces dehydration; and (d) marked decrease in the intra-abdominal pressure in the postpartum period.

Prevention of postpuncture headache requires: (1) the use of a 25- or 26-gauge needle in carrying out subarachnoid block; (2) avoidance of dural puncture with large epidural needles; and (3) ample hydration of the puerpera with 3,500–4,-000 ml of fluids daily by mouth and intravenously if necessary. The efficacy of prophylactic hydration is suggested by the fact that numerous studies have shown that the incidence will be decreased to at least half in patients given fluids compared to those not adequately hydrated (e.g., with a 20-gauge needle, 10% with hydration and 25% no hydration; with a 24-gauge needle, 2% with hydration and 8% without hydration).

Treatment. The first and most important aspect of treatment is psychologic support in the form of explanation of the cause of headache, encouragement, and reassurance that the headache always disappears within a few days. The discomfort of mild headache is relieved with aspirin or other non-narcotic analgesics plus a tight abdominal binder. For a modrate headache, aspirin should be supplmented with 32 or 64 mg of codeine or the equivalent dose of another mild narcotic. If these measures fail and severe headache persists, the patient is administered an epidural "blood patch." This procedure entails indentifying the epidural space, preferably over the site of dural puncture, and injecting 10 ml of homologous blood, withdrawn with sterile precaution by an assistant from a peripheral vein of the patient. A survey of American obstetric anesthetists revealed that over 98% of parturients treated with this method obtained immediate and usually permanent relief.

High or Total Spinal Anesthesia

Very high or total spinal anesthesia and consequent respiratory paralysis may occur as a complication of subarachnoid, caudal, or lumbar epidural block. Following spinal anesthesia, it may be due to an abnormal spread of the therapeutic dose or, more likely, to inadvertent injection of an excessive dose. More frequently, it occurs from accidental injection into the subarachnoid space of large amounts of local anesthetics intended for extradural block. Although in most cases this complication develops within 3–10 minutes of the injection, occasionally it develops as late as 30–40 minutes after dural puncture. Moreover, in some instances, total spinal block has occurred after the initial dose of one or more subsequent injections produced extradural analgesia to about T_{10} as anticipated.

Following such accidental injection, there is a rapid descent of analgesia, and the patient becomes restless, dizzy, drowsy, and dyspneic. Because of the rapid diminution of alveolar ventilation, the patient's voice becomes impaired and finally she cannot speak, develops apnea, and may lose consciousness. For early diagnosis, it is absolutely essential that the patient be closely observed and frequently tested for the level of analgesia, and continuous verbal contact should be maintained.

Preventive measures include aspiration before injection and the use of "test" doses 4–5 minutes before the injection of the therapeutic extradural analgesic dose. Active treatment consists of: (1) artificial ventilation through an endotracheal tube; (2) support of blood pressure with fluids and ephedrine administered intravenously in increments of 5–10 mg; and (3) removal of 15–20 ml of cerebrospinal fluid. The latter can be done by an assistant within 5–10 minutes of the injection before the drug is fixed to the spinal nerve rootlets. Although some clinicians recommend the injection of saline to irrigate or replace the removed CSF, this carries the risk that it may cause a meningeal reaction.

Urinary Retention

Although urinary retention is often considered a complication of subarachnoid, caudal, or lumbar epidural block, there are no data from well controlled studies supporting this thesis. It is more likely that the retention is due to reflex inhibition of bladder function or injury to the bladder caused by pressure of the presenting part. Treatment consists of catheterization of the bladder.

Neurologic Complications

Aseptic chemical meningitis is a rare complication of spinal anesthesia thought to be due to pyrogens, introduction of foreign bodies, or local toxic effects of the anesthetic. Treatment is essentially conservative and consists of emotional support, pain-relieving drugs, and ample fluids.

Bacterial meningitis as a sequel of dural puncture for spinal anesthesia is extremely rare in modern anesthetic practice. It can be avoided in every case by using strict aseptic technique. Treatment consists of pain-relieving drugs, antibiotics, and supportive therapy.

Neurologic sequelae from spinal, caudal, or epidural anesthesia are even more rare. During the past four decades, millions of regional procedures have been used in obstetric patients without such complications (except for recent reports of complications after chloroprocaine). (See page 89.) The cases reported probably represented errors in technique. These serious complications can and must be avoided by rigidly adhering to basic principles of good regional anesthesia.

Cranial nerve palsies can develop as transient complication consequent to the loss of large amount of cerebrospinal fluid and the traction placed on these nerves by the unsupported brain. Since the abducens nerve is the longest of the cranial nerves, it is the most frequently affected. In order of decreasing frequency, the trochlear, oculomotor, and auditory nerves may also be involved.

Prolonged aggravation of symptoms of cranial nerve dysfunction should be avoided, and treatment consists of those measures used to deal with cerebrospinal fluid deficit. Postspinal headache is not always accompanied by a cranial nerve palsy, but a cranial nerve palsy is usually accompanied by a headache.

Cause for the **isolated peripheral nerve injury,** commonly the peroneal and lateral femoral cutaneous nerves, can frequently be attributed to improper positioning of the legs in the lithotomy position. The sciatic, femoral, or obturator nerve lesions can be produced by stretch or pressure on the lumbosacral trunks from the presenting part or from the forceps. Although there may be a tendency to blame spinal or extradural anesthesia for the complications, a thorough neurological examination and diagnostic electromyography will identify the site of the lesion as central or peripheral and will indicate that in most instances it is unrelated to regional anesthesia.

CHAPTER 9. EXTRADURAL ANALGESIA-ANESTHESIA FOR LABOR AND VAGINAL DELIVERY

This chapter is concerned with the application of extradural (a term synonymous and interchangeable with "epidural" and "peridural") analgesia-anesthesia, which entails the injection of the local anesthetic into the spinal canal but ouside of the dura—the extradural space—to relieve the pain of labor and provide anesthesia for vaginal delivery. Although extradural block can be executed at any level of the spinal cord, to relieve the pain of parturition, the solution is injected either into the lumbar spinal epidural space, so-called spinal epidural block, or into the sacral canal, so-called caudal block, or both. Moreover, although it can be achieved with a single injection, most obstetric anesthetists use one of the techniques that permits repeated injections, the so-called continuous technique. Because of its advantages, extradural analgesia in one form or another has replaced subarachnoid block in many maternity centers (Table 11).

TABLE 11. COMPARISON OF EXTRADURAL BLOCK (EB) WITH SUBARACHNOID BLOCK (SAB)

ADVANTAGES OF EXTRADURAL ANALGESIA-ANESTHESIA

1. Incidence and magnitude of maternal hypotension less because slower onset of vasomotor block→more time to mobilize compensatory mechanisms
2. No postpuncture headache unless dura perforated accidentally
3. Theoretically less risk of neurologic sequelae (rare even with SAB)
4. Theoretically less risk from continuous catheter in extradural space than in subarachnoid space
5. Continuous EB technique permits use of analgesic concentration during the first and early second stage:
   a) Less or no effect on perineal sling → less interference with internal rotation
   b) Better bearing-down efforts

DISADVANTAGES OF EXTRADURAL ANALGESIA-ANESTHESIA

1. Technique more difficult than SAB, requires more skill, precision, and experience to insert needle bevel into extradural space
2. Extent and intensity of block less certain (but use of continuous catheter diminishes uncertainty)
3. Onset of analgesia-anesthesia slower
4. Much more (3–4 times) local anesthetic injected
   a) Fetal and neonatal depression may occur
   b) Greater risk of systemic toxicity
   c) Greater risk of accidental total spinal anesthesia

The various techniques of extradural analgesia-anesthesia currently used in obstetrics are as follows:

Spinal epidural block

1. *Standard block* $(T_{10} - S_5)$
   a. Single dose: 2nd/3rd stages
   b. Continuous technique: 1st/2nd/3rd stages

2. *Continuous segmental block*
   a. Initially: segmental $(T_{10} - L_1)$ analgesia
   b. 2nd stage: extend to sacral segments

Caudal block

1. Single dose
   a. 2nd/3rd stages only
   b. Late 1st/2nd/3rd stages
2. Continuous technique: 1st/2nd/3rd stages

Double catheter technique

1. Upper catheter for segmental analgesia
2. Caudal catheter for sacral analgesia-anesthesia

SPINAL EPIDURAL BLOCK

During the past two decades, spinal epidural block has been used with increasing frequency for obstetric patients throughout the world but especially in the United States and, more recently, in Great Britain. In those insitutuions where it is used extensively by properly trained obstetric anethetists, it is considered the ultimate form of obstetric analgesia and anesthesia and is used in most of the parturients with normal, uncomplicated labor. Properly applied (i.e., skillfully executed at the optimal time and with the parturient expertly managed), spinal epidural analgesia-anesthesia provides all of the advantages cited in Chapter 8 and virtually all of the benefits of caudal and subarachnoid (spinal) block without some of their disadvantages. The aforementioned advantages of extradural analgesia over subarachnoid block are particularly applicable to the

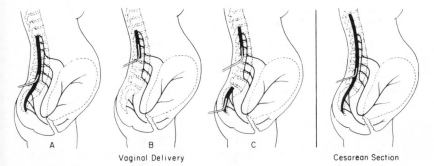

Vaginal Delivery   Cesarean Section

FIGURE 39. Techniques of continuous spinal epidural block used in obstetrics. White tube indicates level of catheter. Black area in spinal canal indicates diffusion of local anesthetic. A, Standard technique for vaginal delivery (analgesia $T_{10} - S_5$). B, Segmental $(T_{10} - L_1)$ block for analgesia during first stage of labor. C, Double catheter technique. For cesarean section, anesthesia is made to extend to T_5. (Courtesy of Bonica, J.J.: *Principles and Practice of Obstetric Analgesia and Anesthesia*, Philadelphia, F.A. Davis Company, 1967.)

spinal epidural techniques. Figure 39 depicts the various techniques of spinal epidural block. Table 12 compares spinal epidural block with caudal block.

TABLE 12. COMPARISON OF SPINAL EPIDURAL BLOCK (SEB) WITH CAUDAL BLOCK (CB)

ADVANTAGES OF SEB

1. Less local anesthetic required
2. Onset of uterine pain relief faster because injection site nearer to uterine sensory fibers
3. Less risk of infection: more difficult to keep skin clean over sacral hiatus than skin over lumbar region
4. No risk of puncturing rectum or fetal head
5. Less anatomic anomalies in lumbar spine than sacrum→less risk of failure

DISADVANTAGES OF SEB

1. Greater risk of dural puncture→more risk of postpuncture headache
2. Greater risk of accidental subarachnoid injection→total spinal
3. Occasional inadequate diffusion to sacral segments → deficient perineal analgesia/relaxation (decrease risk by injecting final dose in Fowler's or sitting position)

An outstanding and very practical advantage of spinal epidural analgesia over both caudal block and subarachnoid block is that it provides a means of achieving specific blockade of pain pathways during each stage of labor. During the first stage, block can be limited to the lower thoracic and upper lumbar segments, thus providing the parturient with relief of pain without interfering with Ferguson's reflex and the cardinal mechanism of internal rotation of the fetal head. During the second stage, spinal epidural block is extended to the sacral segments to provide perineal analgesia (without muscle paralysis) by injecting low concentrations of local anesthetic. After internal rotation takes place, the injection is repeated with higher concentrations of the local anesthetic to produce perineal relaxation, which now is appropriate and beneficial because it facilitates vaginal delivery. When caudal or subarachnoid block is induced during the first stage of labor, it reverses the logical sequence of blockade, producing perineal anesthesia, and, often, relaxation too early in labor at a time when the first is unnecessary and the latter is contraindicated.

It deserves reemphasis that to achieve the stated objective of obstetric analgesia, i.e., good maternal pain relief with little or no risk to the mother or the infant, it is essential for the physician to fulfill the requisites enumerated on page 83. An intravenous infusion should be started well in advance of the block, and a total of 800–1,000 ml of lactated Ringer's solution should be given by the time the block becomes effective. It is preferable to insert the catheter during the latent phase, when the patient is not too uncomfortable. The injection of the local anesthetic to initiate analgesia is made when the cervix is dilated 3–4 cm in multiparas and 4–6 cm in primiparas, contractions are strong, last 35–40 seconds or more, and occur at intervals of 3 minutes or less. The exceptions to these conditions are parturients in whom labor is being induced or stimulated with oxytocin. In such patients, epidural analgesia may be initiated as soon as the patient becomes uncomfortable, because any depressant effects on uterine contractility are obviated by the oxytocin infusion.

Technique

Single Dose Technique. Single dose epidural analgesia-anesthesia is used by some anesthetists and obstetricians because it is simpler and faster to induce, and the puncture with the smaller needle is slightly less traumatic. Its main disadvantage is that it provides less control of the extent, duration, and intensity of the block than is possible with a continuous technique. The injection is made through a 20-gauge or 19-gauge short-bevelled epidural needle inserted in the third lumbar interspace with the patient in the lateral position and using the lack-of-resistance test. If attempt at aspiration in two planes proves negative, 2 ml of local anesthetic is injected as a test dose, and, if no evidence of subarachnoid block is present within 5 minutes, a therapeutic dose of 12–15 ml of local anesthetic is injected. Although in former years, lidocaine was the drug of choice, currently, a solution of 0.5% bupivacaine is preferred because it has no effect on the fetus or the newborn and produces longer analgesia. With the plain solution, it will last for 90–120 minutes, whereas, with the addition of fresh epinephrine in a final concentration of 1:300,000 analgesia is prolonged 20–30 minutes. Therefore, although most clinicians prefer single dose epidural block for the delivery, it can be induced when the cervix is dilated 7–8 cm in multiparas and 9 cm in primiparas with a good likelihood that it will last until completion of the episiotomy repair. To prevent predominant unilateral spread of the local anesthetic, the parturient is made to change to the other side 3–4 minutes after the injection of the therapeutic dose. The management of the patient is the same as described below.

Continuous Technique. Three versions of continuous spinal epidural block can be used for relief or pain of labor and vaginal delivery. The main features of these techniques are summarized in Tables 13, 14, and 15 and Figures 42, 43, and 47. The summary, illustrations, and legends provide an ample overview, and, therefore, only certain pertinent points will be made here. Some experienced clinicians prefer an 18-gauge, thin-walled, Tuohy needle inserted in the midline (Figure 40a), while others prefer the paramedian approach using an 18-gauge, thin-walled, short-bevelled needle (the so-called Crawford point) or a Tuohy needle with a Huber point. The paramedian approach with the Tuohy needle provides the significant advantage of less risk of cutting into the dura with the point of the Tuohy needle and facilitates cephalad advance of the catheter, as depicted in Figure 40b.

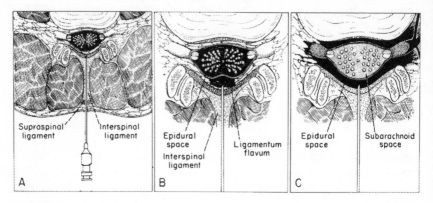

FIGURE 40a. Cross section showing technique of epidural puncture using the midline approach. A, As soon as the point of the needle is felt to enter the ligamentum flavum, an attempt is made to inject saline solution with a 10 ml Luer Lok control syringe. B, As long as the point of the needle is in the ligament there is marked resistance to the injection of the solution, but as soon as the point of the needle enters the epidural space there is sudden lack of resistance. The rapid injection of 5–8 ml of the saline solution mechanically pushes the dura anteriorily away from the needle point. C, Injection of the local anesthetic solution causes it to spread throughout the epidural space, and some eventually enters the cerebrospinal fluid.

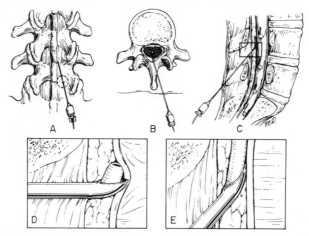

FIGURE 40b. Technique of continous epidural block in the lumbar region using the paramedian approach. A, Posterior view showing relation of site of puncture, direction of needle, and spinous process. Note that the wheal is made 1.5 cm from the midline at the lower tip of the spinous process below the interlaminar space to be entered. The 17-gauge Tuohy needle is introduced so that its axis makes an angle of approximately 15° with the midsagittal plane, shown in B. C, Side view showing the same relation and position of tubing in the epidural space. Laminae and pedicles of vertebrae have been removed. D depicts a Tuohy needle introduced via the midline and advanced sufficiently in the epidural space to partially puncture the dura, and the tip of the catheter is against the dura in an attempt to make a 90° turn cephalad. E depicts the Tuohy needle introduced via the paramedian approach at a sufficient angle to facilitate advance of the catheter into the epidural space. (Courtesy of Bonica, J.J.: *Principles and Practice of Obstetric Analgesia and Anesthesia*. Philadelphia, F.A. Davis Company, 1967.)

Most clinicians prefer the lack-of-resistance test to identify the extradural space. The disappearance of the resistance can be detected by exerting continuous pressure on a 2-ml syringe or preferably a 10-ml Luer-Lok control syringe filled with a solution or air or with a MacIntosh balloon adapted to the needle. Some clinicians prefer to use local anesthetic solutions, others use saline, while others use air. Use of local anesthetics is more hazardous should the needle point unintentionally be advanced into the subarachnoid space and the solution discharged therein. Use of air, because of its compressibility, decreases the sensitivity to pressure changes as resistance and lack of resistance is met. Therefore, saline is best for this purpose (Figure 40a).

Once the bevel of the needle is in the epidural space, the catheter is introduced and advanced no more than 3–4 cm. The catheter is then flushed with 1–2 ml of saline to ascertain it is patent, and then aspiration is attempted to be sure its tip is not in a blood vessel or in the subarachnoid space. This is followed by the injection of 2–4 ml of local anesthetic solution (depending on its concentration) to decrease the risk of accidental total spinal anesthesia. If, after 5 minutes there is no evidence of subarachnoid block, the therapeutic dose is injected (Figure 41).

Some clinicians carry out the injection of the therapeutic dose with the patient in the supine position, with left uterine displacement, and this is maintained for 4–5 minutes, during which time the blood pressure is measured every 30 sec-

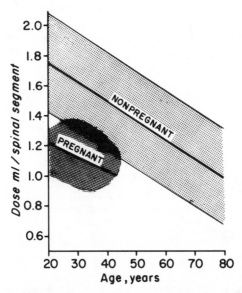

FIGURE 41. Regression lines for dose of epidural solution and age in nonpregnant women and in pregnant women at term. The gravida obviously requires much less (⅔) drug as does nonpregnant patient of the same age. (Modified from and courtesy of Bromage, P.R.; Canad. Med. Assoc. J. 85:1136, 1961.)

onds and, if hypotension develops, it is treated by placing the parturient on her left side. Some clinicians prefer to have the patient in the lateral position during the injection of the therapeutic dose and thereafter, in order to obviate the aortocaval compression. To avoid unilateral analgesia, they inject ½ of the therapeutic dose on one side, and after 3–4 minutes, the patient turns and lies on the other side, and the remaining half of the therapeutic dose is injected (Table 13, Figure 42).

TABLE 13.   TECHNIQUE AND CHARACTERISTICS OF CONTINUOUS STANDARD ($T_{10}-S_5$) EPIDURAL BLOCK

TECHNIQUE	COMPARISON WITH OTHER EXTRADURAL TECHNIQUES
—Needle puncture at L_4→catheter advanced 3 cm (L_3)	**ADVANTAGES**
—Aspiration test and injection of test dose	1. Requires only 1 puncture and insertion of a catheter

—If negative at 5 min, inject 10–12 ml of analgesic dose of local anesthetic → analgesia $T_{10}-L_5$	2. Puncture done in lower lumbar area:
	  a. Less risk of cord damage
	  b. Larger space→easier puncture

—Continuous oxygen and frequent monitoring	3. Provides good analgesia and anesthesia as required
—Top-up analgesic doses as soon as slight pain returns	**DISADVANTAGES**
—Continue analgesia until after internal rotation→inject 10–12 ml of high concentration of LA to relax the perineum	1. Premature numbness of lower limbs during first stage
—If perineal analgesia/relaxation deficient →inject with patient in Flowler's position at least 15 minutes prior to delivery	2. High concentration produces premature perineal relaxation→interferes with flexion and internal rotation
	3. Eliminates bearing-down reflex (but with analgesic dose can push)
	4. Larger doses of drugs required than segmental or double catheter technique

Bupivacaine is the preferred local anesthetic for reasons previously given. If the block is initiated early in the active phase (cervix is 4–5 cm dilated), the 0.25% bupivacaine solution is injected because this is usually effective in relieving pain of contractions of moderate intensity. If, after 15 minutes, the pain relief is unsatisfactory, another therapeutic dose of 0.25% bupivacaine solution is used, and a concentration of 0.5% is injected prior to delivery. As mentioned in the preceding chapter, until recently, 2-chloroprocaine (Nesacaine) has been used and advocated by many obstetric anesthetists because it is hydrolyzed by pseudocholinesterase more rapidly than any other agent, and thus decreases the risk of drug toxicity. The drug is used in 1.5–2.0% concentration during the first stage and 3% concentration for the delivery in order to produce perineal relaxation. Because of the published reports of prolonged sensory or motor deficits

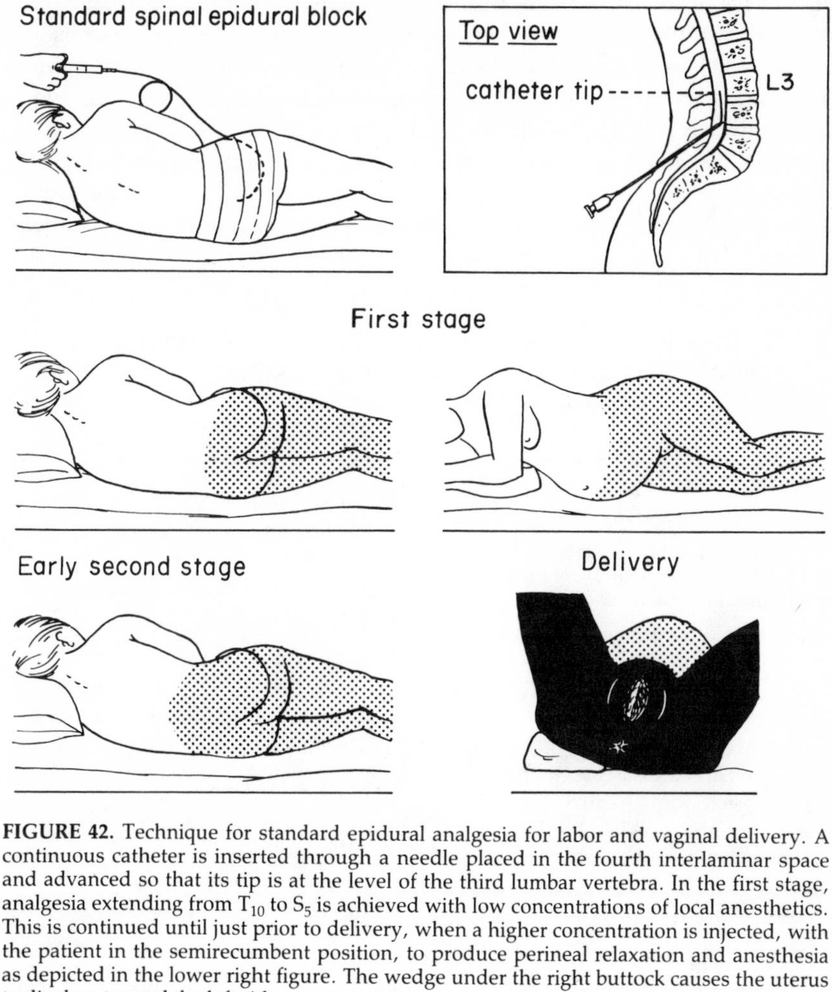

Standard spinal epidural block

Top view

catheter tip ---- L3

First stage

Early second stage

Delivery

FIGURE 42. Technique for standard epidural analgesia for labor and vaginal delivery. A continuous catheter is inserted through a needle placed in the fourth interlaminar space and advanced so that its tip is at the level of the third lumbar vertebra. In the first stage, analgesia extending from T_{10} to S_5 is achieved with low concentrations of local anesthetics. This is continued until just prior to delivery, when a higher concentration is injected, with the patient in the semirecumbent position, to produce perineal relaxation and anesthesia as depicted in the lower right figure. The wedge under the right buttock causes the uterus to displace toward the left side.

and neurologic sequelae, many obstetric anesthetists have discontinued its use. Those who continue to use this agent should take special precautions to avoid inadvertent intrathecal injection. An alternative is to use 0.5% lidocaine (Xylocaine) to produce analgesia for the first stage and early part of the second stage and 1–1.5% lidocaine for the delivery.

The use of low analgesic concentrations of local anesthetic is highly preferable because of the following advantage: (a) less drug is injected and consequently there is less risk of systemic toxicity to the mother and fetus; and (b) there is much less chance of premature paralysis of the lower limbs and perineal muscles. (Premature paralysis of the limbs is annoying to the parturient, while premature paralysis of the perineal sling will interfere with internal rotation and thus increase the incidence of persistent posterior or transverse positions and the necessity for instrumental delivery.) Although with the low concentration the onset of analgesia is somewhat slower, this is more than offset by the aforementioned advantages. An equally effective technique to prevent premature paralysis of the limbs and perineum is to use a single catheter segmental $(T_{10} - L_1)$ epidural block as summarized in Table 14 and depicted in Figure 43. Regardless of the technique used, the parturient should be given oxygen by a nasal catheter or a lightly fitting mask during most of labor and for delivery.

TABLE 14. TECHNIQUE AND CHARACTERISTICS OF SINGLE CATHETER CONTINUOUS SEGMENTAL BLOCK

TECHNIQUE	COMPARISON WITH OTHER EXTRADURAL TECHNIQUES
—Needle puncture at $L_3 \rightarrow$ catheter advanced 3 cm (L_2)	**ADVANTAGES**
—Aspiration test and injection of test dose	1. Requires less drug than the standard technique
—If negative at 5 min, inject 5–6 ml of dilute (analgesic) solution of local anesthetic $\rightarrow$ analgesia $T_{10} - L_1$	2. No effect on uterine contractions
—Continuous oxygen and frequent monitoring	3. No premature numbness of the limbs
—Top-up analgesic dose as soon as slight pain returns	4. No premature perineal relaxation $\rightarrow$ no interference with flexion or rotation
—When pain in limbs and perineum inject 10–12 ml of analgesic concentration with patient in Fowler's position	5. Less effect of local anesthetic on mother and fetus
—After internal rotation inject higher concentration to relax perineum	**DISADVANTAGES**
	1. May produce incomplete analgesia/relaxation of perineum
	2. Requires Fowler's or sitting up position

Usually subjective pain relief starts to develop within 3–5 minutes of injection of the therapeutic dose, and maximal analgesia is present in 12–20 minutes, depending on the drug and its concentration. If there is no evidence of analgesia or at least hypalgesia 10 minutes after the injection of a therapeutic dose, it is likely that the drug was injected outside the epidural space or that it was absorbed too rapidly and block failed to develop. Occasionally, analgesia is present, but not sufficiently high, or is deficient on one side, requiring the injection of additional larger amounts or reinjection with the deficient side down.

Additional "top-up" injections are given as soon as the patient begins to experience discomfort, not waiting until she has severe pain. After the cervix is fully dilated, the mother is coached to bear down voluntarily during each contraction. For optimal results, the patient is asked to grasp her lower thighs with both hands, take a maximum respiration, and then to bear down for 10 seconds, after which she take 2 deep inflations and at the peak of the second inflation, with her lungs filled, she repeats the bearing-down effort. This is continued until the intrauterine pressure nears the relaxation level.

The last injection is given after internal rotation is complete and just prior to delivery, using high concentrations (e.g., 0.5–0.75% bupivacaine or 3% 2-chloroprocaine or 1.5% lidocaine). If perineal analgesia was deficient with previous injections through the single catheter placed high in the lumbar or lower thoracic epidural space, the last dose is injected with the patient in 45° Fowlers position and tilted to the left side.

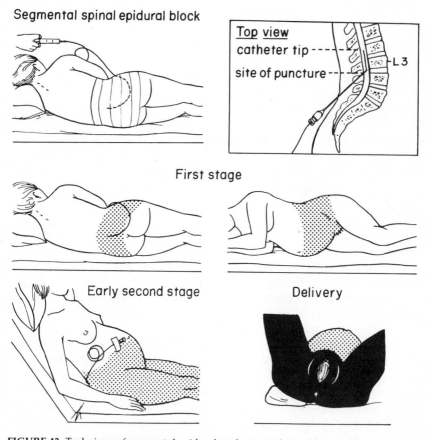

FIGURE 43. Technique of segmental epidural analgesia and anesthesia for labor and delivery using a single catheter introduced into the epidural space and advanced so that its tip is at L_2. Initially small volumes of low concentrations of local anesthetic are used to produce segmental analgesia. For the second stage, the analgesia is extended to the sacral segments by injecting a larger amount of the same concentrations of local anesthetic, with the patient in the semi-recumbent position. After internal rotation, an injection is made of a higher concentration of local anesthetics to produce motor block of the sacral segments and thus achieve perineal relaxation and anesthesia. The wedge under the right buttock causes the uterus to displace to the left.

Management of the Patient. After injection of each test dose and each therapeutic dose, the patient should be observed constantly, and her blood pressure, pulse, and respiration should be measured and recorded every 1–2 minutes. The patient should be made comfortable, reassured, and engaged in conversation, not only for its distracting effect but also to permit the anesthetist to recognize promptly any serious cerebral dysfunction brought about by systemic reaction or hypotension. Since it may take 10–15 minutes for hypotension to develop, it is essential to observe the patient and monitor the blood pressure frequently for at least 20 minutes after each injection and then every 5–10 minutes thereafter. Administration of oxygen is continued until after delivery of the infant.

CAUDAL BLOCK

Caudal block, another form of extradural anesthesia, offers most of the advantages cited for spinal epidural block. Formerly, it was the primary form of regional analgesia for labor and delivery in many clinics, but in recent years it has been displaced by spinal epidural block because of the advantages cited in the proceeding section. Nevertheless, an experienced anesthetist can perform caudal block successfully in up to 95% of patients. Puncture of the sacral canal for caudal block should not be done after the fetal head is on the perineum because of the risk of accidental injection of the local anesthetic into the fetus.

Technique

The technique of caudal block is summarized in Figures 44, 45, 46, and only a few pertinent remarks will be made. The procedure is done either with the patient prone with a 10″ roll under the upper part of the thighs, or, preferably, with the patient on the side in a modified Sims position. In obese patients in whom the landmarks for the sacral hiatus are indistinct, a systematic search is carried out thus: the tip of the coccyx and the spine of the sacrum are identified and a line drawn on the skin. A skin wheal is made 5 cm above the tip of the coccyx, and a 22-gauge spinal needle is used to carry out "exploratory punctures," along the *midline* at intervals of 0.5 cm. (Figure 44). The puncture is first made at the level of the first coccygeal vertebrae, and subsequently cephalad thereto. Penetration of the sacral coccygeal hiatus is easily discerned. When the hiatus has been located, the 22-gauge needle is removed and replaced with the 18-gauge, thin-walled, caudal needle which is advanced about 1 cm beyond the ligament. Although most clinicians advance the catheter only about 3–4 beyond the needle, some prefer to advance it 8–10 cm in order to place its tip at the level of the fifth lumbar vertebrae, because this permits the use of a much smaller volume of local anesthetics (Figure 45). The anatomy of the sacral canal is such that there is a smooth groove in the posterior midline or "roof" of the canal facilitating the cephalad advance of the catheter and minimizing the risk of deviation laterally

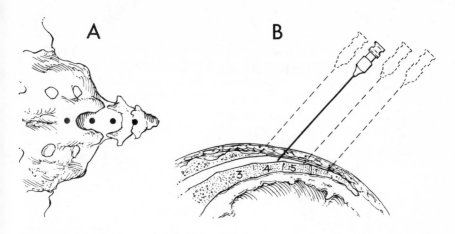

FIGURE 44. Technique of making exploratory punctures to locate center of sacral hiatus as described in the text. A, Posterior view. Dots indicate sites of insertion. B, Sagittal view. (Courtesy of Bonica, J.J.: *Principles and Practice of Obstetric Analgesia and Anesthesia*, Philadelphia, F.A. Davis Company, 1967.)

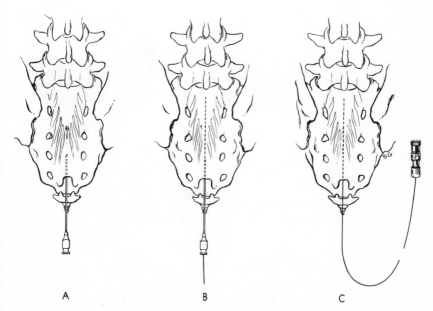

FIGURE 45. Technique of continuous caudal block viewed from behind. A, Special needle in place. B, Vinyl plastic tubing has been advanced to the level of the first sacral vertebra. C, Needle has been removed and end of tubing connected to a Tuohy-Borsch adaptor. (Courtesy of Bonica, J.J.: *Principles and Practice of Obstetric Analgesia and Anesthesia*, Philadelphia, F.A. Davis Company, 1967.)

and into one of the transsacral foramina. Moreover, the internal vertebral venous plexus is sparce in the posterior midline, and the risk of lacerations of veins is very small. Extensive experience also shows that there is little risk of perforating the dura. With this technique, which is actually similar to a low spinal epidural block, only 12–15 ml or ½–⅔ of the usual "caudal block" dose is required. After the catheter is fixed and a test dose has been given, the therapeutic injection is carried out. The management of the patient is the same as described with spinal epidural block.

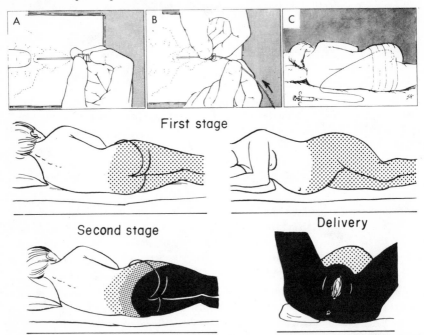

FIGURE 46. Technique of continuous caudal analgesia. The *uppermost figure*, A, shows insertion of a special 18-gauge, thin-walled 7-cm needle through posterior sacrococcygeal ligament. B, The needle has already been advanced 2 cm and its shaft turned 180° so that its bevel faces the roof of the sacral canal, and the plastic catheter is being introduced and advanced 8–10 cm to place its tip at the level of the 1st sacral-5th lumbar vertebrae, as depicted in Figure 45. For the first stage and early second stage, low concentrations of anesthetics are used to produce only analgesia. After internal rotation of the presenting part, a higher concentration is injected to achieve motor block and perineal relaxation (black) and differential block T_{10-12} (light stippling) and lumbar segments (heavy stippling). (A, Courtesy of Bonica, J.J.: *Principles and Practice of Obstetric Analgesia and Anesthesia*, Philadelphia, F.A. Davis Company, 1967.)

DOUBLE CATHETER TECHNIQUE

The double catheter technique entails the insertion of a catheter into the epidural space with its tip at the level of T_{12} vertebra and another placed into the sacral canal with its tip at the level of the third sacral vertebra. These are depicted in Figure 47 and Table 15. The needle puncture for the upper catheter is made at the second or preferably the first lumbar interlaminar space via the paramedian approach and the catheter advanced about 4 cm so that its tip is at the level of T_{12} vertebra. The lower catheter is placed through the caudal needle with its shaft 1 cm within the sacral canal and the catheter advanced 2 cm so that its tip is at S_3 vertebra. The catheters are best inserted at the end of the latent phase or the beginning of the active phase of the first stage when the parturient is not too uncomfortable.

When contractions produce moderate pain and the aforementioned conditions are present (contractions occuring regularly every 3 minutes with an intensity of 30 mm Hg and the cervix dilated at 4 cm in multiparas and 5–6 cm in primiparas), a test dose of 2 ml of the local anesthesia solution is injected through the upper catheter. This dose contains an amount of local anesthetic sufficient to produce a subarachnoid block extending from T_{8-9} to S_5 within 3–4 minutes if the catheter is inadvertently in the subarachnoid space.

If there is no evidence of subarachnoid block, a therapeutic dose of 4–5 ml of 0.25% bupivacaine is injected through the upper catheter. Usually the parturient will have subjective pain relief within 5 minutes of the injection and complete relief in 10–15 minutes. At this time, pin prick testing should reveal a band of analgesia involving $T_{10}-L_1$ dermatomes and sufficient to relieve the pain of uterine contractions. If the analgesic band is not sufficiently extensive, the dose is increased to 6–7 ml to produce a wider segmental block.

When the parturient develops moderate to severe pain in the thighs and eventually the perineum (structures supplied by the sacral segments), 5–7 ml of local analgesic solution (e.g., 0.25% bupivacaine or 0.5–0.75% lidocane) is injected through the caudal catheter. This is usually sufficient to produce pain relief without causing significant motor block, so that the perineal muscles retain sufficient muscle tone for flexion and internal rotation of the presenting part takes place. The caudal injection is repeated to provide analgesia until flexion and internal rotation are complete. Once these are achieved, a caudal injection of 0.75% bupivacaine or, better still, 1.5% etidocaine is injected. The former, and to a greater extent the latter, produce profound perineal muscle relaxation and thus facilitate delivery of the fetus, whether this occurs spontaneously or with the aid of outlet forceps or a vacuum extractor.

The double catheter technique, properly done, is the ultimate in analgesia-anesthesia for labor and vaginal delivery. It provides all of the advantages of regional block without most of its disadvantages. The technique permits exquisitely specific analgesia for the first and second stage and anesthesia for the delivery. The process is accomplished with smaller individual and total doses so that: (1) hypotension and other side effects and the risk of systemic toxic reaction in the mother are minimized; (2) it causes little or no effect on uterine contractions (because of the small doses of local anesthetic); (3) it permits the voluntary use of the abdominal muscles because the analgesic concentrations do not produce motor block; (4) although the caudal analgesia interrupts the afferent limb of the reflex urge to bear down, the parturient voluntarily can exert almost as much increase in intraabdominal pressure as she does reflexively; and (5), most important, with this technique the fetus receives less local anesthetic than with any of the other extradural techniques and therefore incurs no cardiovascular and central nervous system depression.

TABLE 15. TECHNIQUE AND CHARACTERISTICS OF DOUBLE CATHETER TECHNIQUE

TECHNIQUE

—Needle puncture at $L_{2-1}\rightarrow$ catheter advanced 3 cm (T_{12})

—Needle puncture in sacrum at $S_4\rightarrow$ advance catheter to S_3

—Aspiration test and injection of test dose

—If negative at 5 min, inject 4–5 ml analgesic solution of local anesthetic in upper catheter→analgesia $T_{10} - L_1$

—Continuous oxygen and frequent monitoring

—Top-up analgesic dose in the upper catheter as soon as uterine pain returns

—With onset of pain in limbs and perineum inject 5–7 ml of analgesic solution through caudal catheter → analgesia in limbs and perineum

—Continue analgesia until after internal rotation→5–7 ml 0.75% bupivacaine or 1.5% etidocaine via lower catheter → profound perineal muscle relaxation

COMPARISON WITH OTHER EXTRADURAL TECHNIQUES

ADVANTAGES

1. Requires less drug than standard or single catheter techniques

2. The most specific technique for labor and delivery

3. Least effect on mother and fetus

4. No effects on newborn

5. No premature numbness or weakness of limbs

6. No premature perineal relaxation→ no interference with flexion and internal rotation

7. "Rolls-Royce" of obstetric analgesia

DISADVANTAGES

1. Two catheters are required→greater risk of complication and failure

   (Obviated by skilled anesthetist)

EFFECTS OF EXTRADURAL ANALGESIA

Properly executed extradural analgesia provides complete pain relief in 85–90% of patients, partial relief in another 7–12%, and no relief in 2–3%. The relief of pain has beneficial effects on the mother, fetus, and newborn. By blocking the nociceptive afferent input, the block obviates the abnormal reflex responses and the possible complications consequent thereto, mentioned in Chapter 3. Moreover, several clinical studies have impressively demonstrated that complete relief of pain with epidural analgesia during the first stage obviates the metabolic acidosis (reflected by a decrease in base excess and increase in lactate production) that develops in parturients managed with prepared childbirth but given no chemical analgesia or with meperidine or other narcotics (Figures 49, 50). During the second stage, there is a slight time-dependent decrease in base excess and increase in lactate in parturients who have complete pain relief but voluntarily bear down to aid the expulsive efforts of the uterus. On the other

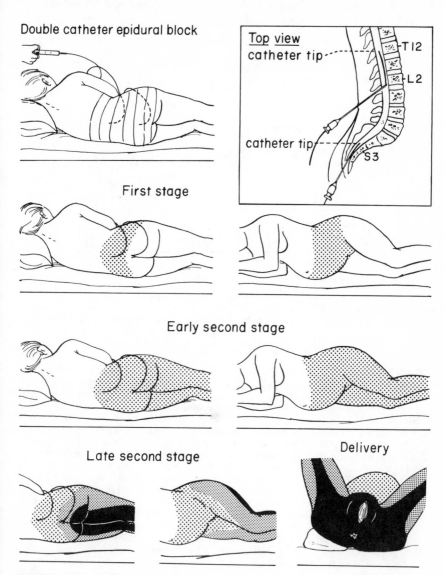

Double catheter epidural block

Top view
catheter tip

T 12

L 2

catheter tip

S 3

First stage

Early second stage

Late second stage

Delivery

FIGURE 47. The double catheter technique for extradural analgesia-anesthesia for labor and delivery. The tip of the upper catheter is at T_{12} and the one for the lower catheter at S_3. As soon as contractions produce moderate pain, small (4–5 ml) volumes of analgesic concentrations of local anesthetics are injected through the upper catheter to relieve the pain. Similar injections are repeated throughout labor. When the presenting part exerts pressure on the pelvic structures and perineum causing pain in the lower lumbar and sacral segments, 5–7 ml of analgesic concentrations of a local anesthetic are injected through the lower catheter. After flexion and internal rotation are completed, a high concentration of the local anesthetic is injected through the lower catheter to produce perineal muscle relaxation and anesthesia of sacral segments (black).

hand, parturients who do not bear down but are delivered with the aid of outlet forceps develop little or no metabolic acidosis.

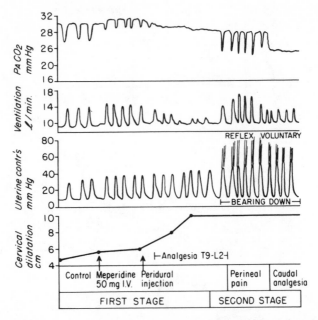

FIGURE 48. Schematic diagram of an actual case showing the relations of cervical dilatation (lowermost panel), uterine contractions, ventilation, and arterial carbon dioxide tension (uppermost panel) in a primigravida managed with narcotic and extradural analgesia. At 5-cm dilatation the parturient had moderate pain and was given 50 mg of meperidine intravenously slowly, resulting in partial relief of pain and consequently smaller changes in ventilation and $PaCo_2$. When the pain became severe, when the cervix was 6 cm dilated, the induction of segmental peridural analgesia had no effect on uterine contractions, but the pain relief eliminated the maternal hyperventilation so that $PaCO_2$ was 28 mm Hg. During the second stage, the perineal distension caused pain and initiation of the reflex bearing-down effort and a concommitant increase in ventilation that caused slight decrease in $PaCO_2$ to about 24–25 mm Hg. The addition of low caudal (L_5-S_5) analgesia eliminated the perineal pain and decreased the respiratory drive. With the voluntary bearing-down efforts, the tidal volume was increased to about 2,500 ml (the inspiratory capacity), but the rate was decreased to 5–6 during the 50–60 second contractions, whereas during the 75–90 relaxation phase, the tidal volume was reduced to 500–600 ml and the rate to 10–12 per minute, so that the average minute ventilation was about 14–16 1/min, resulting in a $PaCO_2$ of 26–30 mm Hg. Compare with Figure 19, page 20.

Effects on Labor

The effects of epidural analgesia on the progress and duration of labor and delivery depend on several factors, including: (a) the condition of the uterine contractions and cervical dilatation at the time the block is initiated; (b) the total amount of local anesthetic injected with each dose; (c) whether or not epine-

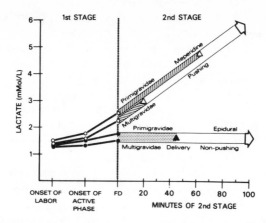

FIGURE 49. Metabolic acidosis and lactate accumulation during labor. ○-Parturients receiving meperidine 100 mg to 150 mg, with no other analgesic during "normal" active labor; ●-parturients receiving continuous epidural analgesia in delivery effected by low forceps but no voluntary expulsive efforts during the second stage; Δ-time of spontaneous delivery in patients receiving meperidine only; ▲-average time of low forceps delivery in patients receiving epidural analgesia. (Courtesy of Bromage, P.R.: *Epidural Analgesia*. Philadelphia, W.B. Saunders, 1978. The curves constructed from data of Pearson and Davis, J. Obstet. Gynaecol. Br. Cwlth. 81:971, 1974.) Compare with Figure 50.

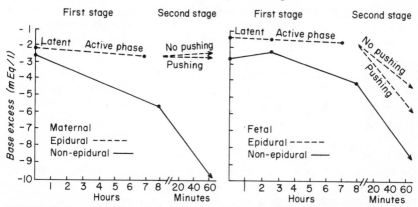

FIGURE 50. Representation of mean changes in extent of maternal (left) and fetal (right) metabolic acidosis during the first and second stages of labor observed in a group of "clinically acceptable ideal" parturients managed without lumbar epidural analgesia and in two similar groups of parturients managed with epidural analgesia, of which those in one group retained a bearing-down reflex and those in the other group did not and were delivered by outlet forceps. Note the significant metabolic acidosis among the nonepidural group of parturients, whereas those given an epidural analgesia experienced little or no change in their acid-base status. Fetuses born of mothers managed without epidural also developed impressive metabolic acidosis during the first stage and an even greater degree during the second stage. Fetuses of mothers given epidural had no change in acid-base during the first stage, but there was a time-dependent increase in metabolic acidosis during the second stage, although the rate of increase was less than in the nonepidural group and least if the mother did not bear down during the second stage. (Modified from and courtesy of Crawford, J.S.: *Principles and Practices of Obstetric Anesthesia*. Oxford, Blackwell Scientific Publications, 1976; based on the data of Pearson and Davis cited in Figure 49.)

phrine is added to the local anesthetic solution; and (d) whether or not oxytocin is used to stimulate or accelerate labor. In patients with spontaneous labor, the induction of standard epidural or caudal anesthesia (T_{10}-S_5) before the aforementioned obstetric conditions prevail is likely to prolong the latent phase by interrupting extrinsic neurogenic influences on uterine contractions. However, the contractions of the late first and second stages are unaffected.

The role of the local anesthetic depends on the total amount (i.e., the concentration and volume). For example, injection of 10–12 ml of 1.5–2% lidocaine or 0.5–0.75% bupivacaine is likely to produce a transient depression of uterine contractions for 8–10 minutes, after which they resume the preinjection intensity, and labor progresses normally. On the other hand, injection of small volumes of the same agents in analgesic concentrations as used with the double catheter technique has no effect on uterine contractions and, in patients with incoordinate or other ineffective contractions, epidural analgesia may *decrease* the duration of the first stage. Since epinephrine may produce myometrial depression, especially if used in amounts larger than 25 µg (5 ml of solution containing 1:200,000 epinephrine), it is best to omit it from the solution. Finally, the use of oxytocin to stimulate or accelerate labor will obviate the myometrial depressant action of local anethetics, epinephrine, and even systemic analgesics and related drugs.

The effect of epidural analgesia on the duration of the second stage is also dependent on several factors. It is well known that the loss of the reflex urge to bear down will significantly increase the duration of the second stage and, if the perineal muscles are paralyzed prematurely, it will double the incidence of posterior or transverse position and the need for "therapeutic" forceps. This is more likely to occur with standard spinal epidural or caudal block using concentrations of local anesthetic that produce partial or complete motor block (Table 10). On the other hand, the use of analgesic concentrations until internal rotation has been completed will permit the parturient to retain sufficient perineal muscle tone so that internal rotation will take place. Moreover, with analgesic concentrations, she retains sufficient abdominal muscle strength and although she has lost her reflex urge to bear down, she is still able to bear down effectively to deliver spontaneously. Even if some muscle weakness or paralysis in the lower limbs develop after a second or third "top-up" dose, the level of motor block with analgesic levels at T_{9-10} is likely not to be higher than T_{12} or L_1. (It has been amply demonstrated that even with 2% lidocaine, the motor block is 3–4 segments below the analgesic level.) However, for the parturient to voluntarily exert sufficient pressure to deliver spontaneously, she should be trained to effectively bear down during the antepartum period and be motivated and coached to bear down during the second stage.

The use of double catheter technique as described above is the best and most effective method of managing the second stage because the anesthetist has much better control of the volume and concentration of the local anesthetic.

Many obstetricians who are not experienced in managing parturients with epidural analgesia have the misconception that it precludes spontaneous delivery and therefore do not use it. Other clinicians use segmental epidural analgesia during the first stage but let it wear off at the beginning of the second stage so that the reflex urge to bear down is retained and the delivery is accomplished spontaneously. This is an unfortunate and indeed indefensible practice because the parturient is deprived of pain relief when she needs it most. Even if the parturient is unable or unwilling to bear down effectively, there is no reason for not using prophylactic or outlet forceps. Indeed, their use has been shown to prove beneficial to both the mother and infant because they shorten the second stage and consequently decrease the maternal work, maternal and perinatal metabolic acidosis, and other risks of prolonged birth asphyxia.

Effects on the Fetus and Newborn

The single catheter standard and segmental techniques and more so the double catheter technique have no deleterious side effects on the fetus and newborn but, rather, have a salutory effect by providing the mother with good pain relief and preventing the aforementioned abnormal reflex responses. On the other hand, the injection of "top-up" doses of lidocaine in 1.5% concentrations for standard epidural block may cause a transient depression of fetal heart beat-to-beat variability, probably reflecting placental transfer of lidocaine. This effect occurs even more frequently and to a greater extent with caudal anesthesia because of the larger amount of drug injected. However, bupivacaine does not seem to have this effect. Therfore, provided the parturient is managed properly so that no aortocaval compression or persistent hypotension occur, the acid-base of the fetus remains stable during the first stage and only decreases moderately during the second stage.

The effects of epidural analgesia with various local anesthetic agents on the Early Neonatal Neurobehavioral Score (ENNS) has been mentioned. It has been reported that newborn infants delivered of a mother who had received standard spinal epidural anesthesia (achieved with a 1.5–2% lidocaine or mepivacaine) had significantly lower scores than infants delivered of mothers with spinal anesthesia or no anesthesia. It has been suggested that this is caused by drug-induced neuromuscular block. In contrast, infants born of mothers managed with epidural analgesia achieved with 0.25–0.5% bupivacaine or with 2 or 3% 2-chloroprocaine had ENNS that were very similar to those in the control (no anesthesia) group. It should be pointed out that the concentrations of lidocaine and mepivacaine used for epidural analgesia were 1.5–2.0%, and the total maternal dose averaged 423 mg and 374 mg respectively given over 2.5–3 hours. Since epidural analgesia can be achieved with 0.5% lidocaine and since 50 mg lidocaine per hour is sufficient to produce highly satisfactory pain relief, it is likely that the incidence of low ENNS can be eliminated with optimal analgesic doses. On the other hand, since it has been shown that even 22–23 ml of 0.75% bupivacaine (168 mg) used for cesarean section do not lower neurobehavioral scores, it must be concluded that this drug is much safer for the newborn, and it explains its current widespread popularity.

SPINAL EPIDURAL NARCOTIC ANALGESIA

The injection of narcotic solutions into the spinal epidural (or subarachnoid) space has been shown to produce profound postoperative analgesia, and some have reported use of this method for labor and vaginal delivery. Although no published reports are available at this time and although the pharmacokinetics of this method have not been elucidated, a summary is presented here because its advantages are likely to cause widespread use. They are: (a) epidural intrathecal narcotics produce analgesia without vasomotor block or without affecting other sensory modalities, (b) this technique produces analgesia for a much longer time (5–20 hours, depending on the drug and dose used) than epidural analgesia achieved with local anesthetics; (c) epidural narcotics do not have deleterious effects on labor; and (d), unless there is a rapid absorption into the maternal blood, epidural narcotics have no effects on the fetus or the newborn. (Several reports of unexpected or delayed respiratory depression in patients managed with epidural narcotics have been published.)

Epidural narcotic analgesia is best achieved by injecting narcotic solution through a 20-gauge epidural needle or via a single catheter or double catheter. For the single dose, injection is made at L_3. A dose of 5 mg of morphine or equianalgesic doses of meperidine (50 mg), methadone (5 mg) or hydromorphone (1 mg) diluted in 8–10 ml of preservative-free saline is injected as soon as the parturient experiences moderate pain. With the double catheter technique, the tip of the upper catheter is at T_{12} and the lower catheter at S_3. As soon as the parturient experiences moderate pain, 2 mg of morphine diluted in 5 ml of saline are injected via the upper catheter. When the parturient begins to have pain in the perineum and lower limbs, 2–3 mg of morphine in 8 ml of saline are injected through the lower catheter. Equianalgesic doses of other narcotics may be used.

Based on the results in postoperative patients, the latency (onset) and duration of analgesia are as follows: morphine 30–40 minutes and 10–20 hours; meperidine 20–30 minutes and 6–8 hours; methadone 20–25 minutes and 4–6 hours; and hydromorphone 12–15 minutes and 8–16 hours. On the basis of these data, it is predicted that a single dose of the particular narcotic should be adequate for the relief of pain throughout the active phase of the first stage and for the second and third stages. Following the injection, the mother should be observed closely for at least 1 hour and at frequent intervals thereafter. If unexpected maternal respiratory depression occurs, naloxone should be given to the mother and repeated until the narcotic-induced depression terminates. Since it has been shown that epidural narcotics do not produce muscular relaxation, an injection of a local anesthetic in concentrations that will produce motor blockade should be made promptly after internal rotation takes place, so that the parturient will have perineal relaxation for delivery.

CHAPTER 10. SUBARACHNOID BLOCK (SPINAL ANESTHESIA)

Subarachnoid block, commonly known as spinal anesthesia, is one of the best methods to produce obstetric pain relief because it is simple to carry out, rapid and certain in its action with a nearly 100% success rate, and, properly administered, produces minimal side effects on the mother and fetus. Two techniques can be used in obstetric patients: standard subarachnoid block, sometimes called *"modified"* saddle block, which is made to extend from T_{10} to S_5 inclusive, and *true saddle block*, limited to the sacral segments to produce perineal analgesia and relaxation. Although modified block is frequently reserved for controlled operative vaginal delivery, it can be used to provide analgesia during the late first stage and second stage. For this purpose, the block is initiated when the cervix is 5–6 cm dilated in multiparas and 6–7 cm in primiparas. By using small doses of tetracaine (Pontocaine) or dibucaine (Nupercaine), analgesia to T_{10} level lasting 2.5–3 hours and perineal analgesia and muscle relaxation lasting 3–4 hours or longer can be achieved. The addition of 200 μg of epinephrine or 2 mg of phenylephrine will prolong these durations by 30–40%. Obviously, this will be very adequate for relief of pain during the active phase of the first stage and second stage and to facilitate vaginal delivery. In the unusual circumstances when the block does not last long enough, it is repeated: there is no valid reason for not doing a second injection, provided these are done with fine needles and without trauma. Many clinicians use hyperbaric lidocaine 25–35 mg in 10% glucose with 200 μg of epinephrine which usually lasts 2–3 hours.

In addition to providing prompt and highly effective analgesia and profound perineal relaxation, subarachnoid block has an important advantage over other regional procedures because it entails the use of such small amounts of local anesthetic which inherently have absolutely *no risk* of systemic toxicity. On this ground it may be considered the regional anesthetic technique of choice when the services of a physician expert in epidural analgesia are not available, and the parturient presents a high risk pregnancy. The disadvantages of the technique include: (a) a small but annoying incidence of postpuncture headache; (b) the fact that it produces marked weakness or paralysis of the lower limbs and the perineum and thus prevents the parturient from moving her lower limbs and interferes with the internal rotation of the presenting part; and (c) most important, the fact that maternal hypotension is more precipitous and of greater magnitude with subarachnoid block than with extradural analgesia, probably because the onset of vasomotor block is so rapid the parturient does not have sufficient time to mobilize compensatory mechanisms. Based on these considerations, the technique is contraindicated in patients with acute or chronic hypovolemia, hemorrhagic shock, or coagulation defects. The premature limb and perineal paralysis is a source of significant dissatisfaction among parturients and obstetricians and has been primarily responsible for limiting its use for the actual vaginal delivery.

Optimal results require careful technique and proper management of the patient, which include: (a) an intravenous infusion of 1,000 ml of fluids prior to the block; (b) the use of very fine (25 or 26 gauge) spinal needles to minimize the incidence of postpuncture headache; (c) the injection of small volumes and doses of local anesthetics to keep the upper limit of analgesia about T_{10}; and (d) rigidly avoiding aortocaval compression. It is well to remember that 2/3 of the dose of a local anesthetic given to nonpregnant women is sufficient. Overdose is the most common cause of maternal deaths (due to "spinal shock") and serious complications that follow induction of spinal anesthesia in pregnant women.

TECHNIQUES

"Modified" Saddle Block

Prior to the induction of anesthesia, an infusion of 1,000 ml of fluids is given at a fast rate so that the entire volume has been administered by the time the block develops. The subarachnoid puncture is made with a 25-gauge needle introduced through the 4th or 3d lumbar interspace using the midline or paramedian approach. Although the sitting position is frequently used to assure that the level of block is limited to T_{10}, the injection can be made with the patient on her side and tilting the table to 15° head-up position before injection (Figure 51). Precautions must be taken to avoid straining or other maneuvers that produce sudden increase in cerebrospinal fluid pressure with consequent excessive diffusion

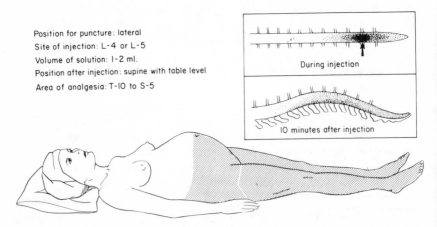

Position for puncture: lateral
Site of injection: L-4 or L-5
Volume of solution: 1-2 ml.
Position after injection: supine with table level
Area of analgesia: T-10 to S-5

During injection

10 minutes after injection

FIGURE 51. Technique of subarachnoid block achieved with the patient on her side and resulting in analgesia extending from T_{10} to S_5. Although the parturient is shown supine for the sake of clarity, after the block is established she should be made to lie on her side during labor and the uterus displaced laterally when she is placed in the lithotomy position. (Courtesy of Bonica, J.J.: *Principles and Practices of Obstetric Analgesia and Anesthesia*, Philadelphia, F. A. Davis, Company, 1967.)

of the agent. Following the successful puncture, a local anesthetic solution containing 3–5 mg of tetracaine (Pontocaine) or 2.5–5 mg of dibucaine (Nupercaine) or 25–35 mg of lidocaine (Xylocaine), diluted to 1–1.5 ml with 5 or 10% dextrose is injected.

Following injection of the drug, the patient lies supine with left uterine displacement, and her blood pressure and heart rate are measured every 30 seconds during the first 10 minutes after the injection and every 3–5 minutes thereafter to promptly diagnose severe hypotension. When the patient is ready to deliver, she is placed in the lithotomy position, and the uterus is promptly displaced to the left, either mechanically or with a wedge under the right hip. If these prophylactic measures are not sufficient and the patient develops hypotension, additional intravenous fluid and small (10 mg) increments of ephedrine are administered intravenously.

Saddle Block

This technique is used to produce perineal analgesia and muscle relaxation. Its indications are similar to those of bilateral pudendal block: it is given to parturients managed during the first stage and early second stage with systemic analgesics, inhalation analgesics, or paracervical block. Since the technique does not entail vasomotor block, it is not associated with maternal hypotension except when analgesia extends higher than intended.

The dural puncture is made with a fine 25-gauge needle introduced through the 4th or 5th lumbar interspace with the patient in the sitting position. One ml of solution made hyperbaric with dextrose and containing 3 mg of tetracaine (Pontocaine) or 2.5 mg of dibucaine (Nupercaine) or 25 mg of lidocaine (Xylocaine) is injected slowly. The patient should be kept sitting for 4–5 minutes after the injection to permit most of the anesthetic to gravitate and become fixed to the sacral nerve rootlets. During the entire period, she should be held by an assistant who prevents her from moving and continuously reassures her. Since in

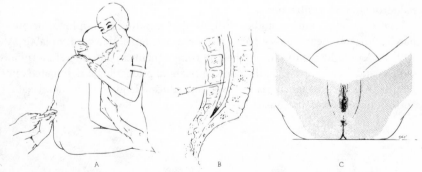

A   B   C

FIGURE 52. Technique of true saddle block. See text for details. (Courtesy of Bonica, J.J.: *Principles and Practice of Obstetric Analgesia and Anesthesia,* Philadelphia, F.A. Davis Company, 1967.)

this position the uterus falls anteriorly away from the vertebral column, it should decrease the risk of aortocaval compression. (Figure 52).

After this period, the patient is made to lie on the side until she is ready to deliver, at which time she is placed in a lithotomy position using the same precautions to avoid the aortocaval compression mentioned in the preceding section.

COMPLICATIONS

The most important complications are discussed in Chapter 7. It deserves reemphasis that all prophylactic measures should be carried out to prevent aortocaval compression and subsequent maternal hypotension. The efficacy of the administration of 1,000 ml of lactated Ringer's solution over a 20-minute period just before the induction of the block and right hip elevation in preventing maternal hypotension has been amply demonstrated. The prophylaxis and active treatment of postpuncture headache is also described in Chapter 7.

SUBARACHNOID NARCOTIC ANALGESIA

The subarachnoid (intrathecal) injection of morphine or other narcotics has been used to relieve acute and chronic pain in humans and during parturition in animals. Like epidural narcotics, this method produces profound analgesia without causing vasomotor blockade or impairment of other sensory modalities. The aforementioned studies have indicated that the subarachnoid approach has the advantage of requiring 1/10th of the dose needed for epidural narcotic analgesia. On the other hand, it has the disadvantage of requiring a dural puncture and the risk of postpuncture headache. Since 0.5–1.0 mg morphine injected intrathecally provides profound analgesia for several hours, it is advisable to inject the narcotics diluted in 2 ml of saline through a 25- or 26-gauge needle introduced in the 2nd or 3rd lumbar interspace. Because of its prolonged duration, the narcotic should be injected as soon as the parturient has moderate to severe pain from uterine contractions.

Well controlled animal studies indicate that intrathecal morphine (or other narcotic) has no deleterious effects on the mother, fetus, newborn, or labor. As with the epidural approach, it is best to complement the intrathecal morphine with a caudal block, true saddle block, or bilateral pudendal block initiated after internal rotation has taken place, so as to produce adequate perineal relaxation and assure complete anesthesia.

CHAPTER 11. PARACERVICAL AND PUDENDAL BLOCKS

Bilateral paracervical block to relieve pain of uterine contractions and bilateral pudendal block to relieve perineal pain during the second stage of labor have been used with erratic frequency in many parts of the world where the services of obstetric anesthetists are not available. This includes hospitals in developed countries, especially those with relatively small obstetric services. Each of these techniques can be administered by the obstetrician and can be used in combination with sedatives, narcotic analgesics, or inhalation analgesia-anesthesia as discussed in Chapters 6 and 12. As with other regional anesthetic techniques, only the summary of the most important points is presented.

PARACERVICAL BLOCK

Although paracervical block was first described and advocated in 1926 by Gerlert in Germany, and a few other reports appeared in the European and American literature, it was not until the mid 1950's that the technique received the serious attention of many obstetricians. As a result of a series of published reports extolling the virtues of the procedure, paracervical block became one of the most popular and frequently used regional techniques during the first stage of labor; it was considered simple and easy to administer by the obstetrician and provided good analgesia in about 70% of parturients and some pain relief in another 10–15%. Moreover, during this initial period of enthusiastic use, the procedure was considered to be the safest method of pain relief for both the mother and infant. However, with extensive experience it became apparent that the technique is not as innocuous as initially thought and it is associated with a number of disadvantages, including: (a) failure rate of 10–30% depending on the knowledge, skill, and experience of the administrator; (b) a small but significant incidence of maternal complications such as mild or moderate systemic toxic reactions and/or transient numbness and sensory disturbances in one or both lower limbs; (c) transient decrease in the intensity or frequency or both of uterine contractions; and (d) fetal bradycardia in 10–30% of cases, depending on the technique and total dose of local anesthetic. A significant number of perinatal deaths and several deaths of gravidas who received paracervical block for therapeutic abortion during the first trimester have been reported. On the basis of published information, the maternal and perinatal deaths were usually due to systemic toxic reactions that were not properly managed.

Fetal bradycardia, the most frequent and most important complication of paracervical block, usually develops within 2 minutes of injection, although it may begin 8–10 minutes later and is due to direct myocardial depression by the local anesthetic. Severe fetal bradycardia is followed by fetal acidosis and then heart rate recovery, and, in extreme situations, by fetal tachycardia. Bradycardia is caused more frequently when there are fetal heart rate abnormalities prior to paracervical block, during repeat blocks, and in association with high risk pregnancies.

Despite a number of animal and human studies, the mechanism for the bradycardia remains controversial. Fetal intoxication by local anesthetic drugs and their metabolites results from direct flow of a high concentration of the drug to the intervillous space. This can be achieved by diffusion of the drug across the uterine artery wall or by direct injection into the artery. Others have suggested that the fetal arrhythmias are the result of acute fetal asphyxia caused by transient uterine artery spasm that, in turn, is provoked by high concentration of the local anesthetic agent in the paracervical region. The larger the dose of local anesthetic the more serious the fetal heart rate changes.

In order to minimize the maternal and perinatal complications, the following guidelines should be adhered to: (1) the procedure should not be started until optimal obstetric conditions prevail; (2) an infusion should be initiated prior to the induction of the block; (3) it is essential to use low concentrations of local anesthetics (e.g., 0.25% mepivacaine, 1.5% 2-chloroprocaine, or 0.5% lidocaine) in volumes ranging from 5–8 ml injected into each side of the parametrium; (4) since it has been noted that the addition of epinephrine to local anesthetic solution increases the severity of the fetal heart rate changes, vasocontrictor should be omitted; (5) the bevel of the needle should not be deeper than 3–5 mm beyond the vaginal mucosa; (6) adherence to basic principles of regional anesthesia including aspiration before injection; (7) the maternal and fetal heart rate should be monitored continuously after each injection; and (8) this technique should *not* be used in parturients with chronic uteroplacental insufficiency or in the presence of preexistent fetal distress.

Technique

With the patient in the lithotomy position, a paracervical block needle with a guard is placed in the lateral vaginal fornix (Figures 53, 54). The guard should prevent the needle point from advancing more than 5 mm beyond the surface of the vaginal mucosa. The injections are made at 4:00 and 8:00 o'clock on the cervical fornix. After careful aspiration for blood, 5–8 ml of local anesthetic solutions is injected on one side. The procedure is repeated on the other side, preferably 8–10 minutes after the first injection in order to decrease the risk of high maternal and fetal blood levels to detect rapid absorption.

The duration of pain relief varies with the local anesthetic and its concentration and total dose and varies widely among different parturients. With 0.25% bupivacaine, relief lasts 75–100 minutes; with 0.5% lidocaine it will last about 60 minutes; and with 1.5% chloroprocaine it will last about 35–40 minutes. Although continuous techniques have been described, the catheters are difficult to keep in place and are not necessary if bupivacaine is used. Following the injections, the parturient is given continuous oxygen, and the fetal heart rate and maternal blood pressure, pulse, and respirations are measured frequently. It is best to have the parturient lie on her side to avoid aortocaval and aortofemoral

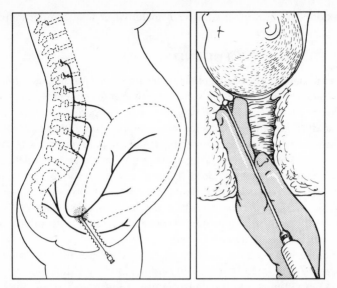

FIGURE 53. Technique of paracervical block. On the left, schematic diagram showing sensory (pain) pathways concerned with parturition and the site of interruption when using paracervical block. The pathways from the uterus, including the cervix, are interrupted, thus relieving the pain of the first stage of labor. On the right, schematic coronal section of vagina and lower part of the uterus showing proper handling of the guide and insertion of the needle. Note that the needle is inserted only a few millimeters beyond the surface of the mucosa. (Courtesy of Bonica, J.J.: *Principles and Practice of Obstetric Analgesia and Anesthesia*, Philadelphia, F.A. Davis Company, 1967.)

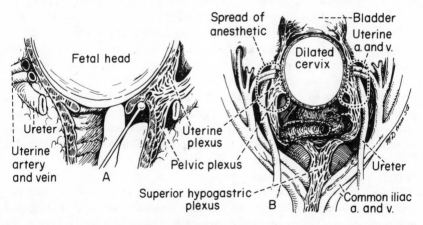

FIGURE 54. *Left*—Enlarged schematic coronal section of lower portion of cervix and upper portion of vagina showing relation of needle to the uterine and pelvic plexuses which are located at 4 and 8 o'clock, whereas the uterine artery and ureter are located at 3 and 9 o'clock. *Right*—Superior view of the pelvis depicting the relative positions of the pelvic plexus and uterine arteries and ureter and the area of diffusion of the local anesthetic. (Courtesy of Bonica, J.J.: *Principles and Practice of Obstetric Analgesia and Anesthesia*, Philadelphia, F. A. Davis Company, 1967.)

compression. The prompt treatment of maternal or fetal complications is discussed in Chapter 8.

PUDENDAL BLOCK

Bilateral pudendal block is an effective technique for producing perineal analgesia and anesthesia during the second stage and for spontaneous or low forceps delivery which stretches the vagina, vulva, and perineum. It also provides anesthesia during the third stage for repair of episiotomy. It affords the advantages of simplicity and ease of administration, it can be given by the obstetrician, and it provides adequate perineal analgesia and, if necessary, muscle relaxation. Skillfully administered, it has no deleterious effects on the mother, fetus, and newborn, or the forces of labor. It is one of the most effective methods to provide perineal anesthesia to parturients whose first stage has been managed with natural childbirth, with sedatives and systemic analgesics, with inhalation analgesia, or with paracervical block.

Disadvantages of the technique are that it is more difficult and time-consuming to execute than low subarachnoid (saddle) block, it is followed by a higher percentage of failures, and it entails the use of much greater amounts of local anesthetics. However, in contrast to subarachnoid block, there is no risk of vasomotor blockade, and there is no risk of maternal hypotension.

Technique

The transvaginal approach is far better than the older transperineal technique because it permits easier palpation of the ischial spine and the sacrospinous ligament which are the important deep landmarks (Figure 55). The type of needle guard as described for paracervical block is used to prevent advance of the needle point more than 1 cm beyond the mucosa. The needle point is made to pass through the sacrospinous ligament, near its attachment to the ischial spine. As soon as the point of the needle is in the ligament, an attempt is made to inject a small amount of saline. As long as the point of the needle is in the ligament there is some resistance to the injection but this promptly disappears as soon as the point of the needle passes through the ligament. When this occurs, the needle is arrested and 5–8 ml or even as much as 10 ml of local anesthetic solution are injected. Since the area where the solution is injected is not as vascular as the paracervical region, the total dose of local anesthetic can be increased moderately.

By using the same concentration for pudendal block as recommended for paracervical block, the risk of maternal and fetal systemic toxicity is minimal, provided, of course, that an attempt at aspiration of blood is negative prior to the injection of the solution. Technical errors include accidental intravascular injection with consequent systemic toxicity and block of the sciatic nerve if the needle is advanced too far posteriorly. The transperineal approach is used only when the presenting part is already very low in the pelvis, making insertion of the palpating hand and needle into the vagina difficult. The care of the parturient is similar to that discussed in connection with the paracervical block (Figure 56).

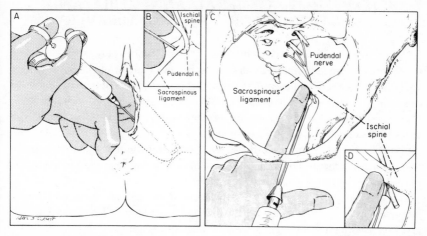

FIGURE 55. Pudendal nerve block. A, The transvaginal approach that entails palpation of the distal spine and sacrospinous ligament with the second and third fingers of the left hand and insertion of the needle with the right hand (for a right-handed individual). B, Enlargement of the injection site. Note that the pudendal nerve passes just posterior to the junction of the tip of the ischial spine and the sacrospinous ligament. The needle is in the sacrospinous ligament, which is used as an important landmark. With the bevel of the needle in the ligament there is resistance to the injection of saline solution, but, as the bevel passes through the ligament, there is sudden lack of resistance, indicating that the needle point is right next to the nerve. C, a superior view of the pelvis showing how the index finger is used to direct the needle point as it approaches the ischial spine. In this instance, the needle is passed posterior to the ligament. (Modified from and courtesy of Bonica, J.J.: *Principles and Practice of Obstetric Analgesia and Anesthesia*, Philadelphia, F.A. Davis Company, 1967.)

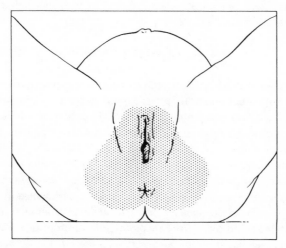

FIGURE 56. Area of analgesia produced using pudendal nerve block. This is usually sufficient to relieve perineal pain during the second stage of labor and for repair of an episiotomy. (Courtesy of Bonica, J.J.: *Principles and Practice of Obstetric Analgesia and Anesthesia*, Philadelphia, F.A. Davis Company, 1967.)

127

CHAPTER 12. GENERAL ANALGESIA AND ANESTHESIA FOR VAGINAL DELIVERY

Despite the usefulness, safety, and increased popularity of regional anesthesia for obstetrics, inhalation anesthetics and other systemic drugs used for general analgesia-anesthesia still play an important role in the relief of pain of childbirth. In many hospitals with small obstetric services, anesthetic personnel skilled in regional analgesia-anesthesia are not available, and, consequently, inhalation or other forms of general anesthesia are used. Moreover, balanced general anesthesia has become recognized as the safest method for the management of parturients with specific obstetric conditions such as hypovolemia and those unusual parturients who refuse a regional technique.

This chapter is devoted to a brief discussion of the optimal application of inhalation analgesia to relieve pain of labor, and of inhalation and "balanced anesthesia" for vaginal delivery. The term, *analgesia*, implies the use of low concentrations of inhalation anesthetics that are sufficient to provide partial and, at times, complete relief of pain and still allow the parturient to remain awake, cooperative, and with her protective laryngeal reflex intact, thereby minimizing the risk of maternal aspiration and causing little or no depression in the mother or newborn. The term, *anesthesia*, implies loss of maternal consciousness with its attendant risks of aspiration and cardiovascular and respiratory depression. Inhalation anesthesia is achieved with a higher concentration than necessary for inhalation analgesia. *Balanced anesthesia* is a term that implies the use of a combination of agents in such a fashion as to exploit their therapeutic efficacy while at the same time minimizing their side effects. In general, inhalation analgesia is used to relieve severe pain of the active phase of the first stage and that of the second stage of labor, and anesthesia is reserved for the actual delivery.

BASIC CONSIDERATIONS

For proper administration of inhalation analgesia and anesthesia, it is essential to consider a number of important physiochemical characteristics of these agents and how their uptake and distribution is affected by changes in maternal ventilation and cardiovascular function, (discussed in detail in Chapter 1). It deserves reemphasis that alterations in ventilation, lung volumes, and cardiac output markedly influence the rate of induction and change in depth of, and emergence from, inhalation analgesia or anesthesia. The analgesic or anesthetic state is primarily determined by the tension of the drug in the brain, which in turn is determined by its tension in the alveoli. The alveolar concentration of inhalation anesthetics is determined by: (1) the inspired concentration of anesthetic gas or vapor, which is regulated by the anesthetist; (2) the rate of replacement of lung air by the anesthetic mixture; and (3) the uptake of the anesthetic by pulmonary blood (Table 16). Lung air washout by the administered gas is determined by alveolar ventilation and the functional residual capacity (FRC) of the lung. With a constant inspired concentration of the inhalation agent, alveolar tension is determined by the balance between anesthetic input through ventilation and anesthetic loss through removal by the pulmonary blood. An increase in alveolar ventilation speeds up the rate of rise in alveolar anesthetic concentration during the induction of anesthesia and hastens anesthetic elimination at the end of anesthesia. Increased ventilation is less important with the less soluble gases such as nitrous oxide and cyclopropane than it is with the soluble agents such as methoxyflurane, trichloroethylene, diethyl ether, chloroform, halothane, or enflurane. A reduced FRC accelerates the rise of alveolar concentration during induction and decreases it at the end of anesthesia. This effect is greatest with less soluble gases and least with the highly soluble agents.

TABLE 16. FACTORS THAT DETERMINE INHALATION ANESTHETIC GRADIENTS

A. **FACTORS THAT DETERMINE ALVEOLAR CONCENTRATION**

1. Inspired concentration
2. Effective alveolar ventilation
3. Functional residual capacity (FRC)
4. Uptake of anesthetic by the pulmonary blood

B. **FACTORS THAT DETERMINE THE UPTAKE OF ANESTHETIC BY THE PULMONARY BLOOD**

1. Alveolar concentration
2. Blood solubility of the anesthetic
3. Cardiac output (pulmonary blood flow)
4. Alveolar-blood anesthetic tension gradient
5. Ventilation-perfusion ratio

C. **FACTORS THAT DETERMINE DISTRIBUTION AND UPTAKE OF ANESTHETIC INTO THE TISSUE**

1. The blood flow per unit volume of tissue
2. The arterial-tissue tension gradient
3. Tissue solubility of the anesthetic
4. Rate of diffusion across the tissue membrane

D. **UPTAKE OF THE ANESTHETIC BY THE BRAIN**

1. Cerebral blood flow
   a. Mean arterial pressure
   b. Vascular resistance: $PaCO_2$, pH, blood viscosity, and intracranial pressure
2. The blood-brain barrier
3. Solubility of the anesthetic in brain tissue

E. **UPTAKE OF THE ANESTHETIC BY THE FETUS**

1. Uteroplacental (intervillous space) blood flow
2. Umbilical blood flow
3. Intervillous-fetal blood concentration gradient
4. Placental membrane (blood-placental barrier)
5. Solubility of the anesthetic in fetal blood relative to maternal blood
6. Fetal cerebral blood flow
7. Blood-brain barrier of the fetus
8. Solubility of the anesthetic in fetal brain

Factors that determine the uptake of anesthetics by the pulmonary blood include: (1) the solubility of the agent in blood relative to gas; (2) cardiac output (pulmonary blood flow); (3) the alveolar-blood anesthetic tension gradient; and (4) ventilation-perfusion ratios. Removal of the agents from the alveoli by the blood is enhanced by greater solubility, higher cardiac output, and lower tension of the anesthetic in the mixed venous blood returning to the lungs. In parturients, the marked increase in alveolar ventilation and decrease in FRC enhances anesthetic uptake while the increased cardiac output enhances anesthetic loss. Usually, the respiratory changes influence inhalation anesthesia much more than the circulatory changes do, so that even with highly soluble agents, the induction of, and emergence from, inhalation analgesia or anesthesia occurs more rapidly in the parturient than in the nonpregnant woman.

Animal and human studies have amply demonstrated that pregnancy, independent of changes in cardiovascular or respiratory function, decreases anesthetic requirement, i.e., the minimum alveolar concentration (MAC*) for a specific inhalation anesthetic in the gravida is lower than in nonpregnant women. In one study, MAC was decreased 32% for methoxyflurane, 25% for halothane, and 40% for isoflurane.

The pattern of uterine contractions must also be understood to properly apply inhalation analgesia or anesthesia. Contractions are usually preceptible by manual abdominal palpation when the amniotic pressure increases at least 10 mm Hg above the normal 10 mm Hg resting tone of the uterus. However, they do not become painful until their intensity is greater than 15 mm Hg, the pressure necesary to initiate cervical dilatation, the primary cause of uterine contraction pain. The intensity and duration of labor pain, therefore, depends on the rapidity and extent of cervical dilatation. This, in turn, is influenced by the frequency, intensity, and duration of each contraction.

INHALATION ANALGESIA

Inhalation *analgesia*, produced by the administration of appropriate concentrations of inhalation agents, is a very effective and widely used method of relieving childbirth pain. This method is usually reserved for use when sedatives and narcotics are no longer effective in relieving moderate to severe pain of the active phase of the first stage and during the second stage. The only exception to this rule is a vaginal examination during the latent phase, when the contractions are not so painful but the examination itself is a very uncomfortable procedure and for which inhalation analgesia serves admirably. It is particularly useful in home deliveries and in hospitals where the services of obstetric anesthetists are not available. This method offers the following advantages: (1) in relation to their

---

* MAC, the minimum alveolar concentration at which nociceptive stimulation produces no reflex responses in 50% of the patients.

respiratory depressant effects, inhalation agents are more potent analgesics than narcotics, and therefore, are much more effective in relieving severe pain of late first and second stage labor, provided they are properly administered; (2) since little metabolism or accumulation occurs, they permit better control of action and reversibility of effect, and can be retrieved from both mother and infant; (3) the mother remains conscious, with full muscle power and protective reflexes, and she can use her auxiliary forces to facilitate the progress of labor; (4) no clinically significant respiratory depression or other adverse effect occurs in the mother, fetus, or neonate; (5) uterine contractions and the progress of labor are unaffected.

A number of careful clinical trials have shown that the fetal acid-base status and oxygenation values remain normal and that the percentage of depressed newborns is similar to that of control groups delivered with local perineal anesthesia. Even when continuous cyclopropane or methoxyflurane analgesia was used for up to 60 minutes, the incidence of neonatal depression was not increased. If inhalation analgesia is used for delivery, a pudendal block should be performed to achieve perineal anesthesia and relaxation.

Although most of the commonly employed inhalation anesthetics are suitable for analgesia in obstetrics, halothane is not recommended because of its low analgesic efficacy. Moreover, although diethyl ether analgesia (achieved by open-drop method or with a machine) has been used for over a century and is still used in some centers, its irritating effects make it less desirable than other agents. Chloroform, the first agent to be used in obstetric analgesia, is now considered potentially dangerous and is rarely used. (The only exception is in special situations in tropical countries where open-drop analgesia is the only method available.)

The agents in current widespread use are nitrous oxide (N_2O), methoxyflurane (Penthrane), and trichloroethylene (Trilene). Enflurane (Ethrane) in concentrations of 0.25–1.25% in oxygen has been shown to be safe and effective as a continuously administered analgesic for vaginal delivery. Apparently its use is not associated with neonatal depression or maternal or newborn renal dysfunction, nor is there any greater blood loss than with other inhalation analgesics. Because there is some risk of the patient losing consciousness during inhalation analgesia, with consequent decrease or loss of protective reflexes, it is advisable to give her 20–30 ml of antacid 15–20 minutes before the inhalation analgesia is started.

Each of these agents may be administered intermittently during each uterine contraction, or continuously. During labor, the agent can be given by the anesthetist or can be self-administered by the patient herself, provided she is closely observed. During delivery, administration by the anesthetist is preferred.

Intermittent Administration

The efficacy of intermittent administration of inhalation analgesia is dependent upon: (1) the latency of analgesia (i.e., the interval between the beginning of administration and the development of sufficient gas tension in the central nervous system to produce pain relief); and (2) the interval between the onset of uterine contractions and the beginning of pain. The latency of analgesia is dependent on the rate at which alveolar concentration approaches the inspired concentration, which, in turn, is dependent upon alveolar ventilation, solubility of anesthetic, cardiac output, and inspired concentration. With 80% nitrous oxide and 20% oxygen, the analgesic latency is about 30 seconds; whereas, with 50% it is much slower. Moreover, the interval between onset of contraction and the onset of pain is 20–30 seconds in early labor and about 10–15 seconds in late labor. For maximum pain relief, it would be desirable to begin the administration of inhalation agents about 20–30 seconds before the onset of contraction so that sufficient gas tension in the brain could be achieved by the time the contraction intensity reaches 15 mm Hg, the level at which pain occurs. The onset of uterine contractions as discerned manually through the abdominal wall must be used to properly time the start of inhalation analgesia administration.

Clinical studies have established that for intermittent administration, the optimum concentrations of inhalation agents are: 40–60% nitrous oxide in oxygen; 0.35–0.5% trichloroethylene; 0.35–0.5% methoxyflurane; and 0.5–1.0% enflurane. These can be considered equianalgesic concentrations, although methoxyflurane and enflurane are somewhat more effective. Several studies in which the lower concentration of nitrous oxide, trichloroethylene, and methoxyflurane were compared revealed no significant difference among the three agents; 50% of parturients derived satisfactory analgesia, 20% derived partial relief, and 30% derived no benefit. With the use of the higher concentrations, nitrous oxide and methoxyflurane were found to provide satisfactory analgesia in 65–70% of parturients, while enflurane produced satisfactory analgesia in 80% of parturients. Nitrous oxide and methoxyflurane, when adminstered together in concentrations lower than those used when either agent is given alone, result in greater incidence (90%) of analgesia and a higher incidence of amnesia than one can achieve by the administration of each agent by itself. Progressive accumulation of methoxyflurane does not usually occur during the intermittent administration of 0.35% but does occur with trichloroethylene. Some patients who inhale 70% nitrous oxide intermittently become semiconscious and excitable. A concentration of 60% nitrous oxide or lower may be preferable if close supervision cannot be provided.

Self-Administration. Patients who are to be managed by self-administration of inhalation analgesia intermittently should be instructed on the proper use of the apparatus. It is important to emphasize proper fit of the mask to the parturient's face so that room air does not dilute the inspired gas mixture. The parturient is also instructed to palpate her abdomen and is given a stopwatch to ascertain the time of onset and duration of each of several contractions and the intervals between the onset of contraction and the onset and duration of the pain. Although the intervals between contractions and the duration of contractions are not the same, especially during the first stage, by averaging the time intervals of several contractions, the parturient is able to predict roughly the onset of the contraction and of the pain.

A variety of equipment is available for self-administration. The Entomox apparatus, available in Great Britain, uses a premixed gas containing 50% nitrous oxide and 50% oxygen. Methoxyflurane and trichloroethylene can be self-administered best by using a demand-flow technique, and several simple devices are available for this purpose that permit the patient to inhale a mixture of the anesthetic and air through a unidirectional valve system without rebreathing. These include the Decota Mark VI Inhaler and Emotril Automatic Inhaler for the adminstration of trichloroethylene, both of which permit inhalation of 0.35 volume % or 0.5 volume % in air. It is possible by the appropriate distribution of tubing and a hood to entrain a supply of oxygen into the inspiratory parts of the apparatus. The Cyprane Inhaler permits the administration of trichloroethylene or methoxyflurane. The Cardiff Inhaler permits the administration of methoxyflurane in a concentration of 0.35 volume % in air. The Penthrane Analgizer is a simple piece of equipment for the administration of methoxyflurane. Because many individuals dislike the application of a face mask, the Cardiff group has developed a mouthpiece that can be adapted to a delivery system instead of the face mask. This simple device has apparently markedly increased the incidence of "patient acceptability" of inhalation analgesia.

For self-administration of inhalation analgesics during the first stage, the patient applies the mask or the mouthpiece to her face and begins breathing very deeply as soon as she discerns the very start of the contractions, which, as previously mentioned, occurs 20–30 seconds before the contraction intensity reaches 15 mm Hg above tone, at which point, the cervix begins to dilate and pain is experienced. If the parturient breathes deeply, the uptake of the inhalation agent by the lungs and thence the blood during the 20–30 second interval between the onset of contraction and the onset of pain is sufficient to increase the gas tension in the brain sufficiently to produce an analgesic effect. She continues to breathe deeply until the end of the painful contraction, at which time she removes the mask and remains relaxed until the next contraction. If the interval between the onset of contraction and the onset of pain is shorter than 20–25 seconds or if for other reasons the patient does not derive relief during the first several contractions, it is advisable to increase the concentration of the inhalation agent to the aforementioned upper values (i.e., N_2O 60% and trichloroethylene and methoxyflurane 0.5 volume %). This is continued until she experiences analgesia, after which time, the weaker mixture is used.

During the last part of the first stage and during the second stage, the technique of intermittent administration must be changed because of the change in the characteristics of uterine contractions and the associated pain: the interval between the onset of contraction and the onset of pain decreases to 15 seconds and later to 10 and even 5 seconds; the pain is more intense and lasts until near the very end of the contraction; the duration of the contraction and of the relaxation phase are both about 100 seconds; and they occur more regularly. Therefore, optimal relief is achieved by instructing the parturient to apply the mask or the mouthpiece 20–30 seconds before the start of each contraction and to continue to breathe deeply until the end of the contraction. When the reflex urge to bear down begins, she is coached to apply the mask or mouthpiece 30 seconds before the beginning of the contraction and to hyperventilate as fast and as quickly as she can for 3 breaths and then to take a 4th even bigger breath and bear down forcefully with the contraction for as long as she can and for at least 8–10 seconds. She is coached to then take another 2 very deep breaths and bear down. This sequence is continued until the contraction ends or she becomes drowsy, at which time she removes the mask (or it falls off her face) and relaxes until the next contraction begins. During the second stage, parturients using self-administered analgesia will require supervision, coaching, and encouragement to ensure effective and safe relief of pain and effective bearing-down efforts.

Intermittent Administration by the Anesthetist. Intermittent administration by an anesthetist can produce even better analgesic effects because he can regulate the concentration of the inhalation agent according to his clinical judgment and the patient's response. After making certain that the parturient has received the oral antacid, that the blood pressure, pulse, and respiration have been checked, and that intravenous infusion has been started, the anesthetist palpates the abdomen during a 6–7 minute period to accurately measure (with a stopwatch) the onset and duration of contractions, the interval between the onset of contraction and the onset of the pain, and the duration of pain as well as the duration of the relaxation phase. If the characteristic profile of the contractions and pain appears to be regular, the inhalation analgesic is administerd about 20 seconds before the contraction. If the contractions are irregular, the inhalation mask is applied at the very onset of the contraction, and a mixture of 70% nitrous oxide in oxygen or 0.5% methoxyflurane or the higher concentration of one of the other inhalation agents or, better still, a combination of nitrous oxide and methoxyflurane is used. The latter takes advantage of the "second gas effect" and thus produces more rapid and more intense analgesia than that produced by either agent used alone. If nitrous oxide is used, it is desirable to administer 100% oxygen at high flow rates of 10 L/min for about 15 seconds before the predicted start of the administration of the inhalation analgesic, and the patient is asked to breathe deeply to wash out nitrogen from the lungs.

The aforementioned mixture of analgesic agent is then introduced, and the patient continues to breathe deeply for 6 breaths taken during the course of 20 seconds, and then she is coached to breathe the analgesic mixture normally until contraction ends.

During the second stage, the mixture of inhalation analgesics is introduced 30 seconds before the predicted time of the contraction, and the pattern follows the same breathing sequence described above. It is important for the anesthetist to continuously reassure and coach the patient and maintain continuous verbal contact to evaluate the level of mentation. If the patient becomes confused, drowsy, excited, or uncooperative, the inspired concentration is lowered. After termination of the contraction, the analgesic is shut off and the patient is made to breathe 100% oxygen for about 15 seconds. As previously mentioned, because this procedure does not provide sufficiently intensive analgesia to obviate perineal pain or the pain of an episiotomy, it is highly desirable for the obstetrician to carry out a bilateral pudendal block for the delivery.

Continuous Administration

Continuous administration of inhalation agents permits maintenance of a more even concentration in the blood and brain and thus provides more effective and more stable analgesia, particularly during the second stage. Although the continuous technique may be used in the labor room, it is more convenient (and more common) to use it in the delivery room where the parturient is transferred during the latter part of the first stage when the intensity and frequency of the uterine contractions increase markedly. Initially, the lower concentration of the aforementioned inhalation analgesics is used, such as 50% nitrous oxide in oxygen or 0.3% trichloroethylene or methoxyflurane or 0.35% of enflurane in oxygen or a mixture of 40% nitrous oxide and 0.25% methoxyflurane in oxygen. These concentrations are gradually increased until their maximum concentration is reached, at which time, the patient should experience good analgesia and still remain oriented and cooperative. As with the intermittent administration, the anesthetist must continuously encourage, reassure, and coach the patient and maintain constant verbal contact. If the patient becomes confused, drowsy, or uncooperative, the concentration is decreased. During the second stage, the patient is coached to take deep breaths as previously mentioned.

The greater efficacy of the continuous technique over the intermittent technique has been demonstrated by numerous studies that indicate, for example, that satisfactory analgesia is obtained by 40–50% of parturients when either nitrous oxide in oxygen or methoxyflurane in oxygen is given intermittently, whereas, each of these agents, given continuously, increases satisfactory analgesia to about 60–65%. A mixture of methoxyflurane and nitrous oxide in oxygen, given intermittently, produces satisfacory analgesia in 60% of parturients, and this is increased to nearly 90% when the mixture is given continuously. It deserves reemphasis that the goal of continuous inhalation analgesia is to provide an optimal analgesic state while maintaining maternal cooperation and consciousness.

GENERAL ANESTHESIA

General anesthesia for normal uncomplicated vaginal delivery can be achieved by administering a single potent inhalation agent or by a combination of inhalation and intravenous drugs—so-called balanced anesthesia. Regardless of the technique used, production of unconsciousness in obstetric patients carries three serious risks: (1) pulmonary aspiration of gastric contents; (2) depression of the newborn; and (3) impairment of uterine contractility with slowing of labor or postpartum hemorrhage, or both. Aspiration of gastric contents remains the most common cause of anesthetic-related maternal mortality. The propensity for vomiting and regurgitation is increased during labor, and the volume of maternal gastric contents may be quite high, regardless of the interval since the last oral intake. In most parturients, the pH of these contents is quite low (less than 2.5). Aspiration of this acid material may result in a fulminant chemical pneumonitis (Mendelson's syndrome). In addition, gastric emptying time is markedly delayed during labor, further increasing the risk of maternal regurgitation and possible aspiration. General anesthetics relax the cricopharyngeal and gastroesophageal sphincters and eliminate the laryngeal and other protective reflexes. Furthermore, some inhalation agents stimulate the vomiting center. To minimize the risk of maternal aspiration, prophylactic measures are followed. These include: (1) oral antacid (magnesium tricylicate or glycopellate) administration, 15–20 ml every 2 hours throughout labor and 30 ml 10–15 minutes prior to induction of anesthesia; (2) rapid, smooth induction of anesthesia; (3) avoidance of any measure that would increase intragastric pressure; (4) the application of cricoid pressure (Sellick's maneuver) with the induction of anesthesia to prevent silent regurgitation; and (5) prompt tracheal intubation.

Maternal and fetal asphyxia is another important hazard of general anesthesia in obstetrics. The parturient is particularly prone to develop hypoxia and hypercarbia if respiratory obstruction, breath holding, or hypoventilation occur. Adequate preoxygenation prior to the induction of anesthesia and careful maintenance of a patent airway are essential for prevention of hypoxia/hypercarbia.

General anesthetics themselves may adversely affect the fetus or newborn directly by placental transfer and consequent fetal depression or indirectly by impairing maternal ventilation, circulation, uterine blood flow, or uterine contractility. All general anesthetics cross the placenta rapidly. Fetal and neonatal central nervous system depression is dose-dependent and time-related; the higher the concentration of inhalation anesthetic and the longer the duration of anesthetic administration, the greater the incidence and degree of neonatal depression. A single sleep dose of thiopental (not exceeding 150 mg) or methohexital (Brevital) (not exceeding 75 mg) or propanidid (not greater than 300 mg) is safe, but larger doses or repeated injections lead to an increased incidence and severity of neonatal depression. In addition to these direct drug effects, the infant is influenced by changes in maternal oxygen and carbon dioxide tensions. Hypoxia of the mother is immediately reflected in a dangerous decline in the oxygenation of the fetus. Maternal hypercapnia leads to fetal carbon dioxide retention. Severe maternal hypocapnia from excessive controlled ventilation impairs fetal oxygenation by causing uterine vasoconstriction and shift of the maternal oxygen dissociation curve to the left, thereby impairing the release of oxygen from blood to maternal tissues and fetal blood. Moreover, if excessive controlled ventilation increases intrathoracic pressure, it will reduce maternal venous return and cause hypotension. Maternal hypotension consequent to deep general anesthesia with halothane results in maternal and fetal acidosis from a fall in uteroplacental blood flow.

General anesthetics have a variable effect on uterine contractility and tone. The less potent inhalation agents, such as nitrous oxide, as well as intravenous barbiturates used to induce anesthesia and skeletal muscle relaxants produce no clinically signifcant effect. In contrast, all potent inhalation agents studied thus far depress uterine activity in direct relation to the depth of anesthesia. However, the degree of uterine inhibition varies with the individual agent. Halothane, diethyl ether, and chloroform produce the most profound uterine relaxation; cyclopropane appears to be the least effective; while methoxyflurane and fluroxene are intermediate in their effect on uterine activity.

Certain conditions pertaining to anesthesia decrease or eliminate some of the deleterious effects of general anesthesia. Small doses of intravenous induction agents (e.g., single doses of 2–3 mg/kg thiopental and 0.4–0.5 mg/kg ketamine) produce little or no fetal/neonatal depression. Moreover, using 40% nitrous oxide-oxygen supplemented with 0.5% halothane produces better analgesia, increases uterine blood flow, causes little or no fetal depression, and no unpleasant awareness by the mother without increasing blood loss from decreased uterine tone. Increasing the maternal arterial oxygen tension to 300 mm Hg or higher increases fetal blood oxygen tension, saturation, and content and results in a better clinical condition of the newborn (Table 19, page 164).

BALANCED ANESTHESIA

The basic technique of balanced anesthesia has proved safe and effective for both mother and newborn. Premedication is generally avoided except for atropine in a dose of 0.6 mg intramuscularly or intravenously. Prior to induction, all of the aforementioned procedures should be carried out, including the oral antacid administration, starting intravenous infusion, and left uterine displacement with a mechanical device or with a wedge under her right hip. About 5 minutes before the induction of anesthesia, the parturient is given 100% oxygen at high flows by mask and an intravenous injection of 3 mg of d-tubocurarine or 1 mg of pancuronium to prevent fasciculation from the subsequent succinylcholine.

Anesthesia is then induced with the following rapid sequence: a single dose of 0.4–0.5 mm/Hg ketamine followed immediately by a single dose of 2–3 mg/kg thiopental and 100 mg succinylcholine while cricoid pressure is applied. Once paralysis develops, an endotracheal tube is inserted, the cuff is inflated, and the adequacy of the inflation ascertained. At this stage, the cricoid pressure is released and the obstetrician informed that he may begin. A *light* plane of inhalation anesthesia is then maintained with 40% nitrous oxide combined with 0.5% halothane or 0.25% methoxyflurane or 0.5% enflurane in oxygen. Of these, halothane is best because it increases uterine blood flow. Following completion of delivery and repair of episiotomy, the inhalation agent is rapidly eliminated to effect a prompt emergence from anesthesia, and the patient is extubated.

KETAMINE

Ketamine, producing so-called "dissociative anesthesia," has been utilized as the sole analgesic-anesthetic agent for vaginal delivery and as an induction agent for cesarean section, followed by 50% nitrous oxide in oxygen and muscle relaxants. Maternal cardiovascular function and uterine blood flow are well maintained. Although some clinicians have used doses ranging from 1–2 mg/kg, these produce serious side effects, including maternal hypertension, respiratory depression, hallucinations, marked increase in uterine tone, emergence delerium, neonatal depression, and hypertonicity.

Ketamine, administered in a single "low" dose of 0.25–0.5 mg/kg, produces intense maternal analgesia without loss of consciousness or impairment of protective pharyngeal or laryngeal reflexes, without effects on maternal cardiovascular function, uterine blood flow, or uterine tone, and with no neonatal depression and only mild maternal dream-like states. Ketamine can also be given in intravenous increments of 10 mg repeated at intervals of 3–5 minutes, with a total dose not to exceed 50 mg over a 30-minute period. With this schedule, analgesia develops in less than 30 seconds and is maintained without loss of consciousness, and the patient is responsive but not infrequently amnesic. Used in this fashion, it is particularly effective for parturients in whom imminent vaginal delivery of the fetus is expected or for parturients with "spotty" regional analgesia for vaginal delivery.

For cesarean section anesthesia, ketamine in a single intravenous dose of 0.-4–0.5 mg/kg followed immediately by thiopental in small doses for induction of balanced anesthesia provides the following advantages: (a) low doses have little neonatal depressing effects; (b) ketamine produces maternal analgesia and amnesia during the induction-delivery period; and (c) the maternal blood pressure and pulse are maintained at near normal levels when the combination is used.

PART C. ANALGESIA-ANESTHESIA IN THE PRESENCE OF COMPLICATIONS AND FOR OPERATIVE OBSTETRICS

CHAPTER 13. MEDICAL AND OBSTETRIC COMPLICATIONS

Pathologic conditions associated with pregnancy and coincidental maternal diseases pose special problems that need to be considered in providing analgesia-anesthesia to the parturient. The scope of this brochure and space limitations preclude consideration of all the complications that may be encountered in clinical practice. The following conditions will be considered in this chapter: toxemia of pregnancy, diabetes mellitus, obesity, heart disease, and fetal complications, including prematurity and fetal distress.

TOXEMIA OF PREGNANCY

Toxemia of pregnancy* is among the most important problems in obstetrics because it accounts for a large number of maternal and perinatal deaths. This condition, peculiar to human gestation and characterized by hypertension with proteinuria or generalized edema or both, requires skillful management, including competent anesthetic care. The anesthetist must appreciate the physiopathology, the severity of the toxemia, and the precarious condition of the infant.

Physiopathology

The cause of toxemia remains unknown, but the basic pathologic mechanisms are well delineated and consist of: (1) widespread arteriolar spasm with consequent decrease in blood flow and varying degrees of tissue hypoxia; (2) retention of water and sodium over and above that retained in normal pregnancy; and (3) imbalance of the coagulation/fibrinolysis system, with a tendency to the evolution of disseminated intravascular coagulation (DIC) with consequent depostion of fibrin localized to certain areas of the vascular compartment, particularly the placental, renal, and pulmonary circulation. The vascular changes, together with local hypoxia of the surrounding tissue, may produce hemorrhage and necrosis. These pathologic mechanisms affect all major organ systems, but a de-

---

* "Toxemia of pregnancy" is a term that has fallen into some disfavor because there is no evidence of a "toxin." It is currently known as "EPH gestosis," although the older term is still used, and in Great Britain the abbreviation "PET" (for preeclampsic toxemia) is still employed.

creased perfusion and impairment of the function of the kidneys and uteroplacental unit are the most important.

Toxemia is classified into 3 types, depending on the severity of the pathology and symptomatology. In *mild preeclampsia* there is usually edema of the lower limbs and mild hypertension. *Severe preeclampsia* is characterized by elevation of blood pressure above 160 mm Hg systolic and 110 mm Hg diastolic, a daily urinary protein excretion of 5 g or more, oliguria, cerebral or visual disturbances, or development of pulmonary edema. *Eclampsia* is characterized by tonic and clonic convulsions that are often sudden and severe and may progress to coma. Some patients pass from severe preeclampsia to coma without convulsions. These physiopathologic changes involve mother, placenta, fetus, and the forces of labor.

Maternal Changes. In the mother, there is shift of fluid from the vascular to the extravascular compartment even before the onset of clinical symptomatology with a consequent hypovolemia, hypoproteinemia, and decrease in electrolytes, particularly sodium and potassium, and an increase in hematocrit. In general, plasma fibrinogen and plasminogen levels are within the lower ranges of pregnancy, but the platelet count is decreased, partial thromboplastin time is shortened, and Factor VIII in the serum is high, as is the urinary fibrinogen-fibrin related antigen.

Blood flow to the kidneys, uterus, and liver is decreased but cardiac work is increased by augmentation of systemic vascular resistance, blood viscosity, and cardiac output. In severe cases, cerebrospinal fluid pressure is elevated, and the tracheobronchial tree is edematous and contains much secretions. Thus, the functions of all vital organs of the mother are significantly altered. In most countries, toxemia is a leading cause of maternal mortality which is usually due to cerebral hemorrhage, toxemic shock, cardiac arrest from hypoxia or pneumonitis, or from aspiration of gastric contents during convulsions.

Placental and Perinatal Changes

Placental changes include premature aging with syncytial degeneration, fibrin replacement, ischemia, necrosis, and infarction. All of these changes, together with decreased uterine blood flow, produce chronic placental insufficiency. During labor, this is further aggravated by a more marked increase in uterine contractility than in non-toxemic gravidas. The *fetus* is at high risk in toxemia. *Fetal death* before labor begins occurs as a result of gradual placental nutritional failure, while death during labor is usually due to severe asphyxia caused by further impairment of the uteroplacental circulation already compromised by uterine contractions, separation of the placenta, or prolapse of the umbilical cord. *Neonatal death* is primarily due to prematurity which may be related to the toxemia itself or incident to the therapeutic termination of pregnancy carried out by the obstetrician to save the mother. The condition of the *live newborn* depends on the severity of toxemia and the obstetric and anesthetic care. Infants delivered of mothers with mild preeclampsia are usually in good condition. However, if severe antepartal and intrapartal asphyxia due to any of the factors mention was present, the newborn will be severely depressed.

Medical Treatment

The medical treatment of preeclampsia consists of three fundamental facets: (1) bed rest; (2) diet, including regulation of fluid and electrolyte balance; and (3) drugs. Bed rest for most of the day with the gravida lying on her side is important. A high protein diet with limited sodium and sufficient calories is recommended. In patients in whom intravenous therapy is indicated, central venous pressure monitoring is essential. In view of the hypovolemia, a balanced electrolyte solution is the fluid of choice, and in gravidas with severe preeclampsia, the addition of plasma-expander therapy with human albumin has been shown to be most beneficial: circulating blood volume increases, the placental blood flow is improved, depletion of protein is replaced, and urine output is increased, while diastolic pressure and edema decrease.

In regard to drug therapy, there are differences of opinion about the use of sedatives and diuretics. Although phenobarbital and diazepam provide safe and effective sedation for the mother, they may have adverse effects upon the infant and therefore are reserved for gravidas who otherwise would not adhere to the prescribed bed rest. The routine use of diuretic agents is discouraged because they are associated with risk of further blood volume contraction, loss of sodium and potassium, alkalosis, and decreased carbohydrate tolerance. In patients with massive systemic edema or incipient pulmonary edema *mannitol* is used. Although *frusemide* was popular in the past and is still being used by some clinicians, several reports of acute pancreatitis developing after use of this drug have discouraged many clinicians from using it. Because it is a very potent diuretic, if it is used, special precautions must be exercised to avoid precipitate falls in maternal blood pressure consequent to the rapid loss of body fluids.

Chlormepiazole, an anticonvulsant with sedative, hypnotic, and antiemetic properties, has been popular in Great Britain for the specific treatment of preeclampsia, but recent studies fail to show any significant changes in either systemic blood pressure, uterine blood flow, or myometrial tone. This is in contrast with the action of *magnesium sulphate*, an agent that has no sedative action on the central nervous system but depresses the function of the neuromuscular junction and produces vasodilation and reduction in uterine contractility with consequent decrease in blood pressure and increase in uterine blood flow and conductance. However, since magnesium sulphate produces only a moderate or transient decrease in blood pressure, for gravidas with severe preeclampsia and hypertension, it is combined with a more potent hypotensive agent. Currently, hydralazine (Apresoline), propranolol, and alpha-methyldopa are the drugs of choice. Hydralazine acts predominantly by direct relaxation of vascular smooth muscle, methyldopa by depletion of tissue biogenic amines, and propranolol by decreasing ionotropic and chronotropic myocardial activity. Cardiac output and heart rate are increased by hydralazine, but they are reduced by both propranolol and methyldopa. Since all three drugs are transferred rapidly across the placenta, fetal heart rate changes in the same direction as the maternal changes are seen.

For the treatment of severe preeclampsia, continuous extradural block to a level of the 8th thoracic segment to denervate the uterus, kidneys, and adrenals has proved to be a valuable adjunct in patients whose blood pressure does not decrease with conventional methods. Several clinical studies have shown that in gravidas with severe preeclampsia, lumbar epidural analgesia caused an average declne in blood pressure of more than 20%. To avoid severe hypotensive episodes, it is best to extend the block cephalad incrementally and slowly. Since reduction of renal and uteroplacental blood flow is due to a combination of vasoconstriction and deposition of fibrin products, extradural block will not affect the latter but will eliminate the former and thus probably increase blood flow, provided of course that maternal hypotension is avoided. Moreover, by blocking the nerve supply to the adrenals, the pain-induced increase in catecholamine secretion is obviated. Regional blockade is also recommended for the treatment of eclamptic coma because awakening appears to occur more readily, the blood pressure is controlled more easily, urine production is increased, and labor can be induced without restlessness or other reaction to pain.

Eclamptic convulsions must be treated promptly as they rapidly lead to fetal hypoxia as evidenced by severe heart rate decelerations. Therapy is based on the same principles as convulsions from other causes: (1) oxygenation (establishment of airway and intermittent positive pressure ventilation with 100% oxygen); (2) depression of cortical electrical seizure activity (ultrashort-acting barbiturate or diazepam); (3) control of muscular hyperactivity (succinylcholine); and (4) reversal of metabolic acidosis (sodium bicarbonate).

The disease, as well as its treatment, produces special problems with regard to anesthetic management and care of the newborn infant. Anemia is masked by the rising hematocrit. Compensation for the effects of sympathetic blockade following regional analgesia is decreased by hypovolemia, hyponatremia, and the action of antihypertensive drugs and magnesium sulphate. If magnesium has been used in larger doses and oliguria occurs, magnesium toxicity may develop, as the magnesium ion is largely excreted by the kidney. Magnesium toxicity, the loss of all reflexes coupled with respiratory depression, and a progressive fall in blood pressure is reversed readily by intravenous injection of a calcium salt (calcium chloride or gluconate). In addition, magnesium potentiates the effect of muscle relaxant drugs.

Management of Newborns. Newborns whose mothers received phenobarbital for sedation may benefit from enzyme induction with facilitated bilirubin metabolism. In contrast, infants whose mothers were sedated with large doses of diazepam may be hypotonic and unable to maintain their body temperatures. In addition, diazepam competes with bilirubin for albumin-binding sites. Neonates whose mothers received reserpine may have respiratory obstruction from nasal congestion that can be treated simply and effectively by instillation of phenylephrine nose drops. Finally, infants of mothers treated with large doses of magnesium sulphate may develop clinically significant hypermagnesemia wth hypocalcemia; however, fetal magnesium excess does not respond to calcium therapy but necessitates assisted ventilation and gavage feeding until the muscular weakness has subsided.

Anesthetic Management

Mild preeclampsia presents no unusual problems, and with few exceptions any systemic analgesics and anesthetics may be used, but regional analgesia is usually best for the mother and infant. With regional analgesia, the degree of maternal circulatory and cerebrospinal fluid pressure responses to the pain of contractions is minimized, and the danger of significant increases in blood pressure is reduced. The incidence and severity of neonatal depression appears to be significantly lower following regional analgesia as compared with general anesthesia. Provided clotting mechanism is normal, the techniques, in order of preference, are: continuous double catheter extradural block; continuous standard epidural analgesia; continuous caudal analgesia; and subarachnoid block. Paracervical block is best avoided.

Patients with severe preeclampsia and those who have had convulsions present serious problems that require highly skilled and specialized anesthetic management. To recapitulate, one must consider that: (1) hypertensive crises may occur; (2) convulsions may be imminent; (3) the fetus is usually premature and placental function is impaired, often seriously; (4) maternal and fetal hypoxia and hypercarbia, electrolyte imbalance, metabolic acidosis, and other serious disorders are usually present; (5) maternal metabolism is usually augmented so that the oxygen consumption is increased; (6) antihypertensive therapy and sedation likely have been used; (7) maternal liver and kidney function is impaired; (8) there is marked increase in uterine contractility which results in a greater degree of birth asphyxia and high risk of precipitate delivery; (9) there is high risk of premature separation of the placenta; and (10) inadequate pain relief may provoke a further increase in blood pressure and convulsions.

Vaginal Delivery. For the severely toxemic parturient, regional analgesia is usually superior to general anesthesia for vaginal delivery because: (1) it provides maximum analgesia, thus eliminating pain, anxiety, apprehension, and other factors that may excite the patient and increase the risk of hypertension and convulsions; (2) it has no direct effect on the heart, lungs, kidney, and liver; (3) it has no direct effect on the infant; (4) it can be used during the first stage, thus making unnecessary the use of large doses of sedatives and narcotics; and (5) it lowers elevated blood pressure. Of course, to derive these benefits, it is essential that these procedures are applied at the right time, carried out skillfully (using optimal doses of local anesthetics), and that every precaution is taken to prevent toxic reactions, severe hypotension, and other complications. Moreover, care must be exercised in evaluating the clotting mechanism. If there is risk of bleeding, it is best to avoid extradural or subarachnoid block. The parturient should be given oxygen inhalation during the latter part of the first stage and during the second stage in order to improve fetal oxygenation.

Continuous double catheter extradural block is the best all around technique for managing patients with severe preeclampsia who do not have abnormal clotting. Catheters should be inserted as early as possible and analgesia initiated as soon as the patient becomes uncomfortable. It deserves reemphasis that low concentrations of bupivacaine (e.g., 0.25%) in small volumes (4–5 ml) are sufficient to relieve the pain of the early first stage, and only if such concentrations are ineffective should 0.5% be used. In this way, any accumulation because of impairment of liver function is minimized. When the pain extends to the lower limbs and perineum, an analgesic concentration (0.25%) of bupivacaine is injected through the lower catheter. After internal rotation takes place, high concentrations of bupivacaine (0.75%) or 1.5% etidocaine are injected through the lower catheter to produce perineal relaxation. It is hardly necessary to emphasize that epinephrine should be omitted because these patients are especially sensitive to its chronotropic and inotropic effects.

Continuous epidural analgesia using the standard technique is equally effective but involves the use of larger amounts of agents, and there is less flexibility regarding perineal analgesia and relaxation. The same comments can be made about continuous caudal analgesia. If the patient is a multigravida and labor is progressing rapidly, subarachnoid block may be the technique of choice.

Paracervical block is not advisable for the same reason given previously: it has been shown that the technique is associated with a high incidence of fetal depression when used in the presence of uteroplacental insufficiency.

If, for any reason, regional analgesia is contraindicated, inhalation analgesia is used during the first stage of labor and continued until delivery, and this is combined with bilateral pudendal block. The best agents for this purpose are 40% nitrous oxide–60% oxygen with potentiation with 0.5% halothane or 1% enflurane. Methoxyflurane and diethyl ether are not the agents of choice because of their potential deleterious effects on the kidney and liver. An alternative is to give a single dose of 10–15 mg of ketamine intravenously.

Cesarean Section. Although some clinicians suggest that regional analgesia should be used for cesarean section only if general anesthesia is contraindicated, properly executed spinal epidural or subarachnoid block affords the same advantages to the gravida as they do for labor and vaginal delivery. In order to obtain optimal results with regional anesthesia, it is essential to have continuous central venous pressure measurements, adequate hydration with balanced electrolyte solution, and effective left uterine displacement. If the blood pressure declines despite these prophylactic measures, a small dose of ephedrine (10 mg) is injected intravenously and repeated if necessary. However, if the patient has received antihypertensive therapy that renders ephedrine ineffective, a dilute phenylephrine solution should be considered. Oxygen 100% at high flows should be administered by face mask or nasal cannulae until after delivery of the infant.

General anesthesia for cesarean section also requires a balanced electrolyte solution for intravenous hydration. Moreover, if hypertension is severe, a trimethaphan infusion should be on hand to promptly treat a precipitous rise in blood pressure that may occur with endotracheal intubation. The technique of balanced general anesthesia should be used with the sequence described on page 137.

DIABETES MELLITUS

Most problems associated with diabetes mellitus during pregnancy are related to changes in glucose tolerance, alterations in insulin requirement, and a greater liability toward ketosis and acidosis. The need for insulin is progressively increased during the first 2 trimesters, reaching a maximum during the early 3rd trimester with no further change until after parturition when an abrupt decline occurs. The type and amount of insulin required may vary in the same patient at various stages of pregnancy. In addition, the vascular effects of diabetes are often aggravated, and infection and preeclampsia are more frequent. The placenta undergoes premature aging with multiple necroses in the small villi.

Obstetric Care

Pregnancy is usually electively terminated between the 36th and 38th weeks of gestation. Proper timing is guided by serial determinations of serum or urinary estriol levels (indicating fetal jeopardy due to placental insufficiency) and of amniotic fluid lecithin-sphyngomyelin ratios and creatinine levels (indicating fetal maturity). The newborn, despite normal or greater than normal size, should be considered as if premature, as many organs are not fully functional. Maternal blood sugar levels must be determined at regular intervals because they tend to decline rapidly to below normal levels, necessitating intravenous or oral glucose administration.

The patient is admitted about 1 week earlier than the date of planned termination in order to permit careful control of the diabetes. Three days before the anticipated delivery, she is changed from long-acting insulin to regular insulin 4 times a day; the dosage is adjusted to the degree of glycosuria determined in urine samples tested before breakfast, lunch, dinner, and at bedtime. Proper anesthetic care includes rational fluid therapy during labor and parturition. Oral feeding is discontinued the evening before induction of labor, and fluids are administered intravenously at a rate to prevent dehydration and ketosis. It is recommended to alternate 1,000 ml of 5% dextrose in balanced electrolyte solution with 1,000 ml of 5% dextrose in water. During labor, the equivalent of 10 g of glucose is required to compensate for the increased muscle efforts, but salt intake should be limited to 18 g/24 hr. Regular insulin is continued according to urine samples tested at least every 6 hours, but no attempt should be made to maintain the urine completely free of sugar, as the adverse effects of hypoglycemia far outweigh those of mild hyperglycemia. This regimen is maintained if cesarean section becomes indicated because of fetal distress or because induction of labor has not been successful within 48 hours. However, when the cesarean section is performed electively, dextrose and insulin should be withheld until after delivery of the infant, to decrease neonatal glucose imbalance.

Anesthetic Care

The anesthetic management of parturients with diabetes mellitus requires that the anesthetist be fully acquainted with the patient's disease, the present status of the diabetes, the condition of the fetus, the progress of labor, and the plan for medical and obstetric management. From both the maternal and fetal viewpoints, it is essential to use agents and techniques that avoid aggravation of the preexisting disturbances in acid-base and glucose metabolism or impose a further workload on the renal and cardiovascular systems of the mother. Anesthetics that increase endogenous catecholamine release, hyperglycemia, and metabolic acidosis should be avoided because they aggravate the preexisting ketosis. Anxiety, fear, and pain of labor, a tiresome induction of anesthesia, and hypoxia and hypercarbia often aggravate the preexisting ketosis.

As far as the fetus is concerned, it is especially important to remember that: (1) diabetes is associated with premature aging of the placenta and decreased placental blood flow, resulting in chronic placental insufficiency; (2) the infant is frequently premature, extremely delicate, and excessively large; (3) labor may be prolonged, either because of the large baby or imparied uterine contractility or both; (4) the amount of birth asphyxia is usually greater among fetuses delivered of diabetics as compared with those delivered of nondiabetic mothers; and (5) the fetus may have a serious anomaly.

All of these factors can contribute to make the diabetic fetus at risk. Therefore, maternal arterial hypotension, hypoventilation, or extreme hyperventilation from any cause must be avoided. It is best to avoid or use only minimal amounts of systemic depressants that pass the placental membrane and those that will prolong labor and thus increase the hazard of birth asphyxia. The anesthetic should permit a nontraumatic application of outlet forceps or facilitate breech delivery if this is contemplated (although currently cesarean section is preferred to breech delivery). Further impairment of uterine contractility must be avoided.

These conditions are best met with regional analgesia-anesthesia for both vaginal and abdominal delivery because it has little or no effect on the mother, fetus, and newborn, provided of course that the usual precautions to prevent aortocaval compression and maternal hypotension are exercised.

Extradural Block. In skilled hands, the double catheter extradural analgesia technique, described on page 110, is best. The catheters are inserted during the latent phase, and segmental analgesia $(T_{10} - L_2)$ is initiated at the onset of the active phase of the first stage and continued for the rest of parturition to relieve uterine contraction pain. With the onset of pain in the perineum and lower limbs, 6–7 ml of 0.25% bupivacaine are injected through the caudal catheter to produce analgesia limited to $L_{3-4} - S_5$. Analgesia is continued until after internal rotation when the same volume of 0.75% bupivacaine or 1.5% etidocaine is injected to produce adequate perineal relaxation. Continuous spinal epidural analgesia with a single catheter or continuous caudal analgesia using the standard techniques are also effective and safe, provided the amount of local anesthetic used is kept to a minimum and the maternal blood pressure maintained near normal.

Subarachnoid Block. Low spinal anesthesia extending to T_{10} is also a highly effective method to relieve the pain of childbirth in diabetic mothers, provided maternal hypotension is avoided. As previously mentioned, this technique can be initiated when the cervix is dilated 4–6 cm, using dibucaine (Nupercaine) or tetracaine (Pontocaine) to effect prolonged analgesia. If the block wears off before delivery, it can be repeated. True saddle block $(S_1 - S_5)$ can be used to produce perineal pain relief and relaxation for the actual delivery. It is an excellent technique to combine with segmental epidural block or as the terminal anesthetic in parturients who have been managed with sedatives and inhalation analgesia.

Paracervical block should not be used, because the local anesthetic agent may potentiate the effects of chronic uteroplacental insufficiency and produce fetal and neonatal depression. On the other hand, bilateral pudendal block is a useful adjunct to systemic or inhalation analgesia.

General Analgesia and Anesthesia. If, for some reason, regional analgesia-anesthesia cannot be used, inhalation analgesia is used for the latter phase of the first stage and for the second stage and delivery. If analgesia is not adequate, very small doses of ketamine may be used to potentiate the analgesic action. Bilateral pudendal block is used to produce perineal analgesia and relaxation.

OBESITY

Obesity may be defined as an excess of more than 20% over ideal body weight. With such an excess, the incidence of diabetes during pregnancy is inreased 10 times, that of preeclampsia 7 times, and that of pyelonephritis 5 times. Abnormal presentations of the fetus are 2½ times more common than normally. Complications occur in more than 60% of cases, and operative obstetric interference becomes necessary in about 30%.

The obese patient has an increased oxygen cost of breathing but a decreased pulmonary volume because her excess weight has brought about changes in the mechanics of respiration. Her vital capacity is greatly reduced, and enhancement of the elastic recoil of the thoracic wall produces a decrease in the expiratory reserve volume. There is reduced ability to expand the chest during inspiration so that some areas of lung are poorly ventilated and pass inadequately aerated blood into the systemic circulation causing arterial hypoxemia. Hypoventilation may be further aggravated by body positions such as lithotomy or Trendelenburg position that reduce the efficiency of the respiratory musculature. The cardiovascular consequences include a larger circulating blood volume and increased cardiac stroke volume. This, together with a greater resistance of the larger vascular bed, increases the work of the heart, causing ventricular hypertrophy and diffuse myocardial disease. Finally, the fact that fat does not contain as much water as other body tissues may lead to problems in fluid management.

Anesthetic Management

The anesthetic problems are predominantly technical but also concern oxygenation and drug dosage. The technical problems start with difficulty in performing a venipuncture. Regional anesthetic methods pose the difficulty of identification of landmarks and the unpredictability of levels of blockade. For vaginal delivery, a low thoracic subarachnoid block administered in a sitting position is the simplest and safest procedure. However, a continuous epidural block provides better and longer analgesia-anesthesia. It is advisable to use a long (15 or 18 cm) 22-gauge needle to amply infiltrate the subcutaneous tissue, muscle, and periosteum and also to *explore* the position of the lamina and *the ligamentum flavum*. In every obese patient, it is necessary to use a special, long (18 cm) Tuohy needle or short-bevel epidural needle using the midline or preferably the paramedian approach. Having the parturient in the sitting position facilitates identifcation of the midline and the vertebral level. The lack-of-resistance test is used to identify the epidural space. The amount of local anesthetic needed for subarachnoid block is related to the gravida's height and not her weight. Moreover, obese gravidas require smaller volumes of local anesthetic for extradural analgesia than do nonobese gravidas.

With general anesthesia, there are even greater difficulties in maintaining the woman's upper airway because the tongue and oropharyngeal tissues may cause obstruction before the patient can tolerate an oropharyngeal airway, and manual support of the mandible may be all but impossible without causing injury to the skin or facial nerve. Tracheal intubation may be difficult because of the heavy jaw and a short thick neck. Awake intubation is preferred in these patients to avoid any period of hypoxia. Finally, ventilation must be adequately assisted or controlled at all times (preferably by means of a volume-limited ventilator) because descent of the diaphragm is hindered by the fat-laden abdomen as well as the fetus. The dose of systemic drugs depends on lean (not total) body weight, while tissue uptake of inhalation agent is signifcantly determined by the regional blood flow per unit volume of tissue.

HEART DISEASE

The significant improvement in the management of patients with both acquired and congenital heart disease has resulted in an increase in the number of women who become pregnant and require highly skilled anesthetic care. Because painful uterine contractions and bearing-down efforts produce a cumulative increase in cardiac output of about 80% above that of prelabor, complete pain relief and elimination of the bearing-down efforts are among the most important parts of the obstetric and anesthetic management of these patients.

Rheumatic Heart Disease

Rheumatic heart disease accounts for 80–85% of cardiac disease in pregnancy. Mitral stenosis, alone or combined with mitral insufficiency and/or aortic valvular disease, occurs in at least 75% of these patients. Although most of them fall into functional classes I and II, pregnancy and parturition impose significant risks. This is amply demonstrated by several hemodynamic studies in gravidas with various valve lesions, most of whom demonstrated reduced cardiovascular responses to the demands of pregnancy and exercise. This is especially marked in those with mitral stenosis whose cardiac output values are below the mean for normal pregnant women, regardless of stage of gestation or functional class, and show little change from the postpartum values. It is essential that management be directed towards preventing cardiac failure by reducing gestational hypervolemia and minimizing demands for increased cardiac output. During pregnancy, this entails bed rest, sedatives to combat anxiety, restriction of sodium, and use of diuretics. Digitalization may be indicated for its inotropic action or to slow or convert a rapid or irregular ventricular rate. Quinidine and DC cardioversion have been used without harm to the fetus *in utero*.

During labor and parturition, the following measures are recommended: (1)

hydration with a slow infusion of dextrose in water; (2) relief of stress and apprehension by administration of a tranquillizing drug early in labor; (3) complete relief of pain and abolition of bearing-down sensations with regional analgesia; and (4) inhalation of oxygen by face or nasal cannulas. A combined low thoracic-low caudal block by the double catheter technique is best, using the smallest possible amount of local anesthetic to reduce vasodilatation to which the fixed output heart is very sensitive. The technique provides excellent conditions for forceps or vacuum extraction delivery and can be extended to reduce venous return to the heart should cardiac failure with pulmonary edema suddenly occur. In addition, sympathetic blockade can be continued after delivery to reduce the postpartum increase in cardiac work and, then, be reduced slowly over the next 12–24 hours. Hypotension should not occur if the block is executed judiciously and aortocaval compression is avoided. However, if a vasopressor drug should become necessary, one with peripheral-acting properties such as phenylephrine (Neosynephrine) in dilute solution administered carefully to accurately titrate the drug with restoration of the blood pressure is preferable to ephedrine because the latter increases the work of the heart.

Patients who have had a prosthetic valve placed and are on chronic heparinization present a special problem. When labor starts, heparin should be discontinued or its effects antagonized by a calculated dose of protamine so that regional analgesia can be administered without the hazard of extradural hematoma formation. A spinal block given with a fine-gauge needle may be less traumatic than extradural analgesia. Heparinization may be reinstituted 24 hours following delivery. When anticoagulation cannot be adequately reversed, epidural block or subarachnoid block should not be employed, because of the risk of intraspinal hemorrhage. Instead these parurients should be managed with systemic tranquilizers and narcotic administration during the early phase of labor, paracervical block during the active phase, and pudendal block during delivery, using 5–8 ml of 0.25% bupivacaine bilaterally for block techniques. Inhalation analgesia without overbreathing helps the degree of pain relief.

Congenital Heart Disease

Patients with *acyanotic heart disease* such as pulmonic stenosis can be managed with any form of analgesia-anesthesia provided it is properly administered. Episodes of hypotension must be avoided. Paracervical/pudendal block is an excellent combination. Continuous segmental epidural block for relief of uterine pain and low caudal or saddle block for the delivery can be used by skilled anesthetists provided hypotension is avoided. This is especially important in patients with low cardiac output and in those with a history of episodes of syncope or vascular collapse. They are useful in patients with impending or overt right-sided heart failure. Since there is a narrow margin between pulmonary congestion and inadequate cardiac output, hypotension or hypertension must be avoided.

Anesthesia for parturients with patent ductus arteriosus, septal defects, or other forms of *cyanotic heart disease* who are to deliver vaginally must fulfill the following requisites: (1) effective relief of pain throughout labor and delivery; (2) avoidance of even transient episodes of hypotension because they may lead to reversal of the blood flow and further oxygen unsaturation; (3) avoidance of struggling, coughing, laryngospasm, bronchospasm, and other respiratory difficulties during the administration of anesthesia because these aggravate pulmonary hypertension and other physiopathology and may lead to the reversal of shunt; (4) elimination of bearing-down efforts during the second stage because these also further increase right atrial and ventricular pressure and central venous pressure; (5) avoidance of an increase in mean intrathoracic pressure associated with assisted or controlled ventilation; (6) avoidance of hypoxia at any cost; and (7) avoidance of direct myocardial depression.

These objectives are best achieved by using small doses of sedatives and systemic analgesics during the early part of the first stage, *paracervical block* to control uterine pain and bilateral *pudendal block* to provide perineal anesthesia. If paracervical block cannot be used, inhalation analgesia is a good substitute to control the pain of the latter part of the first stage and second stage. True saddle block may also be substituted for bilateral pudendal block. Anesthetists with great experience in the technique can use segmental epidural analgesia limited *strictly* to $T_{10}-L_1$ combined with low caudal analgesia limited to S_2-S_5, taking special precaution to avoid maternal hypotension by carefully administered intravenous fluid load and having the parturient kept on her side.

Congestive Heart Failure

Congestive heart failure is one of the most serious cardiac conditions encountered in anesthetic practice. In administering anesthesia, the primary considerations are to avoid myocardial depression, an increase in the workload of the heart, and marked alterations in blood pressure. Since these patients have marked increase in sympathetic tone and consequent compensatory venoconstriction, care must be exercised to avoid extensive vasomotor block because this will result in serious maternal hypotension with compromise of coronary perfusion. Moreover, large amounts of local anesthetics must be avoided because these may further depress the myocardium.

These requisites are best met with segmental (T_{10}-L_1) epidural analgesia to control uterine pain and true saddle (S_1-S_5) block for the actual delivery. Saddle block avoids the use of large amounts of local anesthetics and the extensive vasomotor block associated with the usual technique of spinal, epidural, or caudal block. The latter techniques can be used, provided low (analgesic) concentrations of local anesthetic are employed. The limited vasomotor block may prove beneficial to the patient with congestive failure by producing a bloodless phlebotomy, thus decreasing the work load of the heart. It is best to give these patients 100% oxygen throughout most of labor.

Cesarean Section

Cesarean section in patients with heart disease is best achieved with balanced general anesthesia because it is associated with less alteration in blood pressure and cardiovascular dynamics and with less psychologic stress than major regional anesthesia. It is especially important to use the smallest possible amounts of thiopental (100 mg) or ketamine (10 mg) because the circulation time may be prolonged and the action of the drug delayed. Balanced anesthesia as described on page 137 is especially indicated in patients with congenital heart disease and parturients with coronary artery sclerosis, hypovolemia, and anemia in whom extensive vasomotor block inherent in subarachnoid or extradural anestheia should be avoided. In patients with severe shunts, it is important to avoid an increase in mean intrathoracic pressure because of the risk of reversing left-to-right intracardiac shunt and thus aggravating the already existing arterial hypoxemia.

FETAL COMPLICATIONS

Prematurity

In considering the optimal anesthesia for the mother, it is essential to remember the characteristics of the premature infant pertinent to anesthetic care that include: (1) greater susceptibility to the respiratory, circulatory, and central nervous system depressant effects of narcotics, sedatives, intravenous, and inhalation anesthetics; (2) greater susceptibility to birth asphyxia and consequently greater degrees of acid-base deviation (metabolic acidosis); and (3) less efficient hepatic and renal function. The greater degree of susceptibility to depressant effects of drugs is probably related to the increase in the blood-brain barrier permeability of these drugs in the fetus and newborn. The relative softness of the fetal skull, the fact that frequently in these cases the mother begins to bear down before the cervix is fully dilated, and the increased frequency of very rapid spontaneous delivery all contribute to potentiate birth asphyxia and increase the risk of perinatal mortality and morbidity.

In view of these considerations, it is best to avoid narcotics and use only small doses of sedatives and psychologic support during the latent phase and to initiate early some form of regional analgesia. Properly applied, regional analgesia-anesthesia is the best method for pain relief in premature labor and delivery. In contrast with narcotics and systemic analgesics, regional analgesia produces complete pain relief without concomitant neonatal depression, provided maternal complications are avoided.

The double catheter technique (described on page 110) provides optimal conditions for delivery of the premature infant. By preventing the bearing-down reflex, relaxing the perineal floor after internal rotation, avoiding the superimposition of metabolic acidosis, and permitting a gentle, controlled delivery, epidural analgesia reduces considerably the perinatal hazards to which the prematurely delivered infant is exposed. The next best technique for these situations is the single catheter standard lumbar epidural analgesia. Although it requires the use of greater volumes of local anesthetics, there will be no perinatal depression if bupivacaine is used in low concentrations. For reasons given on page 100, continuous caudal analgesia is less preferable than continuous spinal epidural block but may be used to advantage, provided low concentration of local anesthetics is used. Similarly, spinal anesthesia can be used for premature labor and delivery, provided prophylactic measures against maternal hypotension are taken. In all instances, in addition to fluids administered to the mother, it is necessary to have her laboring on her side to avoid aortocaval compression.

If, for some reason, regional analgesia is unavailable, it is best to give these patients very small doses of sedatives and use inhalation analgesia to relieve pain. Because the small size of the infant facilitates delivery, inhalation analgesia combined with bilateral pudendal block is adequate, even for the delivery.

Multiple Pregnancies

In selecting the method of analgesia and anesthesia for the delivery of twins, triplets, or even greater multiplicities, consideration should be given to the following: (1) the infants are usually premature and have been exposed to a less efficient placental function during pregnancy than single infants; (2) the infants are likely to be exposed to greater risks of such complications as congential anomalies, toxemia, placenta previa, abruptio placentae, and prolapsed cord; (3) the second infant usually has had less efficient placental function during pregnancy, but more importantly, is exposed to serious risks of severe intrapartal asphyxia from a numer of conditions peculiar to delivery of the second twin; (4) the mother of multiple infants is exposed to increased risk of hemorrhage, toxemia, anemia, as well as aspiration of gastric contents if she has unexpectedly rapid labor after eating a large meal; and (5) the obstetrician may need to change the obstetric management unexpectedly and may require prompt anesthesia for version and extraction, breech delivery, or cesarean section. To plan for all of these exigencies, the anesthetist must be consulted as soon as the patient enters the hospital so that the patient may be seen and properly prepared before the anesthesia is needed.

The anesthetic management of these patients is similar to that described above for premature infants. It is best to prevent the bearing-down reflex, to adequately relax the perineal floor, to carry out a gentle, controlled delivery, and, most importantly,to prevent aortocaval compression. This is important for both infants, but is is especially important with respect to the well-being of the second infant because of the relatively long time that the mother is likely to have spent in the lithotomy position before the second twin is delivered. These conditions are best met with continuous epidural analgesia, preferably by using the double catheter technique for reasons previously given. Provided there is no maternal hypotension, fetal distress is absent, and there is no requirement for an urgent delivery, the extradural analgesia is usually adequate for delivery of the second infant. On the other hand, if delivery of the second twin requires complete uterine relaxation, a rapid induction of balanced general anesthesia as described on page 137 is carried out and 1–1.5% halothane is included in the inhalation mixture for the minute or so that the obstetrician needs uterine relaxation.

Instead of spinal epidural analgesia, continuous caudal analgesia may be used, provided that low concentrations of bupivacaine are used. Similarly, subarachnoid block is effective to produce the aforementioned conditions, and, since it entails the use of very small doses of local anesthetic, there is no perinatal depression, provided maternal hypotension is avoided. Again, it deserves emphasis that the patient must be on the side during labor, and, if the lithotomy position is used for delivery, it is necessary to displace the uterus laterally by placing a wedge under the right hip. The mother should be made to inhale 100% oxygen during the latter part of the first stage and during the second stage and delivery.

Fetal Distress

Fetal distress is defined as a compromise of the condition of the fetus caused by an acute or chronic unfavorable fetal environment. It is usually characterized by marked alteration in cardiac rate or rhythm, in the passage of meconium in the vertex presentation, and fetal acidosis—signs indicating fetal asphyxia. The causes of fetal distress include: (a) *acute decrease in placental blood flow* caused by aortocaval compression, abnormal uterine contractions or hypertonus, severe maternal hypotension, compression of uterine vessels by forceps, manipulation, tumors, etc., and uterine vasoconstricion caused by vasopressors or severe maternal hyperventilation; (b) *acute decrease of the diffusing surface of the placenta* consequent to placenta previa and abruptio placentae; (c) *chronic decrease in placental perfusion* (high risk pregnancy) associated with toxemia of pregnancy, diabetes mellitus, hypertension, postmaturity, and grand multiparity; (d) *compression of the umbilcal cord*; (e) *severe fetal cardiovascular depression* from accidental injection of local anesthetic into the fetus or placental circulation, or gross overdose of general anesthetic; and (f) *maternal complications*, including severe pulmonary hypoventilation, inadequate circulation from shock, cardiac failure, or normovolemic hypotension, and insufficient oxygen carrying capacity as obtains in severe anemia and methemoglobinemia.

Diagnosis of fetal distress requires careful and continuous monitoring of the fetal heart rate and rhythm and the biochemical status of the infant. The limitations of the auscultatory method are now generally recognized and have prompted development of equipment that permits the continuous and simultaneous measurements of fetal heart rate (FHR) and myometrial activity. The FHR patterns that can be observed and recorded are made up of: (a) *baseline changes* that occur in the absence of or between uterine contractions; and (b) *periodic changes* associated with uterine contractions. FHR patterns that suggest fetal distress include such baseline changes as tachycardia (FHR above 160 beats/min) or bradycardia (FHR below 120 beats/min) and such periodic changes as late decelerations, usually indicative of uteroplacental insufficiency, and variable decelerations, usually indicating cord compression. These patterns are illustrated in Figure 57.

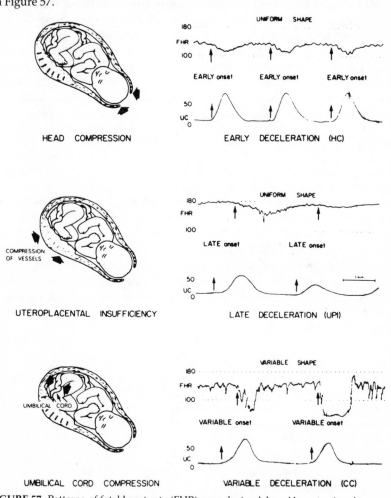

FIGURE 57. Patterns of fetal heart rate (FHR) seen during labor. *Upper tracing* shows early deceleration that occurs during the peak of uterine contractions and is due to pressure on the fetal head; *middle tracing* shows late deceleration due to uteroplacental insufficiency; and *lower tracing* variable deceleration due to umbilical cord compression. Arrows denote time relations between onset of FHR changes and uterine contractions. (Courtesy of Hon, E.H.: *An Introduction to Fetal Heart Rate Monitoring*, New Haven, Harty Press, Inc., 1969.)

155

Fetal heart rate beat-to-beat variability and acceleartion in association with fetal movement are increasingly recognized as indicators of fetal well-being. The oxytocin challenge test (or contraction stress test) is a sensitive indicator of fetal reserve between the 28th and 44th weeks of gestation. Small doses of oxytocin are infused in order to achieve 3 contractions over a 10-minute period. If late deceleration patterns occur, the fetus is considered at risk, while absence of later decelerations indicates a fetus that is in good condition.

Measurement of the pH and other biochemical parameters of fetal scalp blood should be used as another diagnostic criterion in fetal distress and as a prognostic procedure in patients with high risk pregnancies. In the latter group, the first blood sample is obtained when active labor has prevailed for about an hour, even in the absence of fetal distress. In the presence of the normal acid-base state and unchanged clinical signs of distress, a repeat sample is obtained in 1 hour. When the pH is below 7.25, the sample is repeated immediately. If fetal samples show a rapid decrease in pH or if pH is 7.20 or below in 3 consecutive samples, delivery should be carried out as rapidly as possible.

Management. When there are signs of fetal distress, prompt intervention is required. The type and time of delivery should be decided according to the station of the presenting part and dilation of the cervix. If there is evidence of an abnormal FHR pattern and an increasingly severe fetal metabolic acidosis and a poorly dilated cervix, then cesarean section is indicated. From the viewpont of perinatal mortality, the speed and care with which delivery is carried out are important in the prognosis for the fetus. The clinical management of the various etiologic factors of fetal distress is beyond the scope of this volume. As far as anesthetic management is concerned, a rapid delivery requires balanced anesthesia, or spinal anesthesia in the hands of someone skilled to do it with dispatch. The latter technique is contraindicated in patients with severe hypovolemia or hypotension.

CHAPTER 14. ANESTHESIA FOR OPERATIVE VAGINAL DELIVERY

Occasionally, vaginal delivery may necessitate manipulation or instrumentation to effect completion of the second stage of labor. This presents certain potential problems to the unsuspecting obstetric anesthetist. It is the purpose of this chapter to make the obstetrician and his anesthetist colleague aware of the importance of their joint effort to obtain optimal conditions for safe delivery with maternal protection. The following procedures will be briefly discussed: (1) manual rotation; (2) vacuum extraction; (3) forceps manipulation and delivery; (4) shoulder dystocia; (5) breech manipulation; (6) internal podalic version and extraction; and (7) other procedures including manual removal of retained placenta and external cephalic version.

MANUAL ROTATION

The current indication for manual rotation is either minor right occiput anterior or left occiput anterior conversions to occiput anterior, or the obstetrician's decision that an occiput anterior position delivery is preferred to an occiput posterior one (approximately 6% of vaginal deliveries). Manual rotation is most often performed by application of constant pressure to one of the prominent ridges of the overlapping suture line during uterine contractions. This, of course, not only does *not* necessitate uterine relaxation but contradicts it. With adequate uterine and auxiliary abdominal forces, enough pressure on the uterus and fetal head may be exerted by the obstetrician's hand to effect rotation to various degrees.

The procedure may be performed with: (1) no analgesia; (2) simple regional analgesia (paracervical and pudendal blocks); or (3) major regional techniques (lumbar epidural, caudal epidural, subarachnoid block).

The operator may elect not to use analgesia and will rotate by persistent careful manipulation. It is advisable to at least have perineal analgesia achieved with bilateral pudendal block. Some obstetricians prefer a sensory and motor blockade and, therefore choose to have a spinal epidural or subarachnoid block. For such a short simple maneuver, subarachnoid block is probably preferable.

VACUUM EXTRACTION

The primary usefulness of the vacuum extractor is in situations in which the desired fetal position is not as easily attainable or there is need to avoid space occupying instruments in tight pelvic conditions. Properly used, this instrument is safe and serves as a "trial forceps" in mid-pelvic and transverse arrest cases. It may also be used when marked suture line overlap and asynclitism make it difficult to identify the occiput position properly. It should *not* be used to attempt a forced delivery through an undilated cervix. On the other hand, in cases where the cervix is quite flacid and practically eliminated, it may be applied and used successfully to effect further dilatation, descent, and delivery.

Analgesic requirements for vacuum extraction are minimal. The primary objective is the application of the largest cup that can be applied transvaginally to the fetal head without entrapping the cervix or vagina. Analgesia can be achieved with low doses of ketamine or inhalation analgesia. It is preferable that the patient remain conscious, cooperative, and capable of vigorous bearing-down effort to aid in fetal rotation and descent. When the parturient is not cooperative and the obstetrician has difficulty in actual placement of the cervical cup, a true saddle block may be performed for adequate vaginal analgesia and relaxation. Since this blocks only sacral segments, it does not interfere with uterine contractions or the voluntary bearing-down efforts when these are required for descent and rotation of the fetal head. Lumbar epidural, caudal, and pudendal analgesia also produce relaxation of the pelvic diaphragmatic muscles and may be used successfully to aid in ease of application.

FORCEPS MANIPULATION AND DELIVERY

Recent critical appraisal of fetal and maternal trauma subsequent to midforceps delivery have stringently curbed the incident of this procedure; and, in fact, forceps use in general has decreased over the past decade. The reason for this trend is that it has been demonstrated that delivery by cesarean section carries less risk of maternal and neonatal injury and morbidity than vaginal delivery requiring midforceps. Nevertheless, there are probably situations that indicate the use of Kjelland forceps and rotation, the Scanzoni maneuver for rotation from occiput posterior to occiput anterior, and the use of Kjelland forceps or Barton forceps and maneuver for rotation from occiput transverse to occiput anterior.

In determining the optimal method of analgesia and anesthesia, it is essential to evaluate the condition of the patient because many parturients who have required forceps delivery have had a more difficult labor and were therefore more fatigued and probably had greater amounts of accumulated fluids and gas in the stomach. Moreover, the fetus may have been subjected to a greater degree of birth asphyxia which is likely to increase neonatal depression and may be further aggravated by the operative maneuver. Optimal analgesia for these patients should include complete analgesia of the lower uterine segment and vagina and perineal analgesia and muscular relaxation. In addition, it may be necessary to have analgesia of the upper birth canal.

In view of these considerations, regional analgesia-anesthesia is far better than general anesthesia because it provides complete analgesia and relaxation without significant maternal or perinatal depression. The double catheter technique is the best method, but the single catheter spinal epidural block or subarachnoid block provides equally good analgesia and motor relaxation. Pudendal block is usually not adequate for midforceps rotational maneuvers and even when combined with light inhalation analgesia will usually not provide adequate relaxation essential for these maneuvers and concomitant protection of the fetus. In the rare case when uterine relaxation is essential, it would be necessary to administer inhalation anesthesia using a potent uterine relaxant such as halothane as a part of balanced anesthesia as discussed on p. 137.

SHOULDER DYSTOCIA

Shoulder dystocia is of a serious life-threatening consequence to the fetus and presents itself as a sudden, unexpected emergency to the obstetrician. It deserves special attention and sufficient emphasis so that when it does occur both the operator and the anesthetist will act in an efficient and coordinated fashion to effect a safe, controlled delivery that is also painless.

The classic patient profile for shoulder dystocia is a multiparous patient who experiences a prolonged period of descent through an extended second stage with a fetus of estimated weight in excess of 4,000 g and who receives pudendal block or local analgesia for delivery. The incidence of this problem is small (less than 2% of fetuses greater than 4,000 g) but it is associated with a perinatal mortality of near 16%. The situation develops for the unsuspecting obstetrician after delivery of the head and is recognized by immediate retracion of the head toward the perineum as the wide shoulder girdle becomes wedged in an anterior-posterior direction behind the symphysis pubis. The dilemma deepens as the operator realizes that he cannot effect delivery unless undue pressure is exerted upon the fetal head and concomitantly on the brachial and cervical plexuses. Complete delivery must be achieved immediately because the face becomes rapidly cyanotic.

The idea analgesia for shoulder dystocia entails analgesia of the birth canal and perineum and relaxation of the pelvic musculature. Spinal epidural, caudal, or subarachnoid block are all suitable to achieve these conditions. However, in those instances in which the parturient has wedged the shoulder more tightly into the pelvis, any further attempt to deliver the posterior arm may only cause greater maternal distress and involuntary pushing responses. Under such conditions, the anesthetic of choice is a "crash induction" and maintenance with inhalation analgesia as described on page 137. It must be stressed that, as soon as tracheal intubation has been achieved, the obstetrician should begin delivery of the posterior shoulder, since the muscle relaxant succinylcholine will provide immediate profound pelvic muscular relaxation.

BREECH PRESENTATION

Breech presentation occurs in 3% of full term and 5% of premature deliveries.

There are four types of breech presentation: (1) frank; (2) complete; (3) incomplete; and (4) footling. Presently, all of these except the frank presentation are considered best managec by cesarean section delivery. The rationale behind this is that the frank breech is the only type that affords an adequate dilating wedge of sufficient diameter to the cervix to produce adequate cervical dilatation and simultaneously protect the umbilical cord from prolapsing during dilatation, descent, and rotation. However, even vaginal delivery of a frank breech is associated with increased maternal and perinatal morbidity, because of prolonged labor, the stress of manipulation, and tearing of the perineum. The increased perinatal morbidity in term infants is due to cord compression, trauma during delivery, and aspiration of amniotic fluid, blood, or meconium if the infant gasps before delivery of the head. In addition, immature infants presenting as breech are subjected to a combination of trauma and birth asphyxia that produces neonatal depression.

The primary life-threatening condition to the fetus is entrapment of the fetal head after the delivery of the small diameter pelvic girdle and shoulders. This so-called "ice cream cone effect" is particularly a threat in premature neonates where the head is not moulded and its size is proportionately greater than the shoulder or pelvic girdle size. Under these circumstances—incomplete cervical dilatation—there is a prematue urge to bear down, with further risk of trapping of the head by the incompletely dilated cervix.

To minimize the aforementioned risks and provide the parturient and her fetus with optimal anesthetic care, it is essential for the anesthetist and the obstetrician to communicate, coordinate, and cooperate. The best anesthetic technique for breech delivery is continuous double catheter epidural analgesia. This permits the use of minimal amounts of local analgesic agents during labor and permits the injection of either 0.75% bupivacaine or, better still, 1.5% etidocaine through the lower catheter to produce complete perineal relaxation. By relieving pain, preventing the bearing-down reflex, relaxing the perineum, avoiding metabolic acidosis, and permitting gentle, controlled delivery, epidural analgesia reduces considerably the perinatal hazard to the infant delivered by breech. Single catheter continuous epidural analgesia is also useful but requires greater amounts of local anesthetics. The same comments can be made about continuous caudal block which has been used with good results. Spinal anesthesia is also a useful procedure.

In the event that extensive intrauterine manipulation is necessary, rapid induction of balanced general anesthesia as described on page 137 is carried out and 1–1.5 halothane is included in the inhalation mixture to produce myometrial relaxation for the brief time required by the obstetrician. As soon as the head is delivered into the lower birth canal, the halothane is discontinued and rapidly eliminated by mildly hyperventilating the patient. This not only causes a shorter emergence but, more importantly, also decreases the amount of blood loss from uterine atony.

INTERNAL PODALIC VERSION AND EXTRACTION

Internal podalic version and extraction is rarely used because cesarean section produces much less maternal and perinatal morbidity. Version and extraction has been associated with uterine rupture, cervical and perineal laceration, hemorrhage, and puerperal sepsis. Nevertheless, under optimal conditions of uterine relaxation and full cervical dilatation, internal podalic version and extraction may be used in the management of second twin with fetal distress. This requires skillful administration of general balanced anesthesia with halothane included to produce rapid and profound myometrial relaxation for the brief period needed by the obstetrician. All prophylactic measures are performed for the protection of the mother to prevent aspiration of gastric contents into the lungs. Once the manipulation is completed, inhalation anesthesia is rapidly eliminated by mildly hyperventilating the parturient.

OTHER PROCEDURES

The operation of *manual removal of retained placenta* can be accomplished under either continuous epidural or spinal anesthesia with ease and without causing discomfort. Although it is widely believed that general anesthesia is needed to produce uterine relaxation, regional analgesia is preferred because it obviates the danger of aspiration of gastric contents and other side effects of general anesthesia. Usually, the obstetrician has no difficulty in inserting his hand through the cervix in order to extract the placenta. If spinal epidural, caudal, or subarachnoid block analgesia is unavailable, a combination of bilateral pudendal block and paracervical block will provide adequate analgesia and acceptable operating conditions.

Most obstetricians who practice *external cephalic version* believe it should be attempted without anesthesia so that they may detect possible rupture of the uterus. On the other hand, there are those who believe that the addition of general anesthesia to provide uterine relaxation enhances success of the procedure, but, general anesthesia carries the risk of causing partial detachment of the placenta. Moreover, if version cannot be performed successfully while the patient is awake, it is likely that the infant will reassume its position as a breech presentation after having been manipulated under general anesthesia. Again, in most of these instances, it is far better to deliver the infant by cesarean section than to attempt these maneuvers.

CHAPTER 15. ANESTHESIA FOR CESAREAN SECTION

Currently, cesarean section is being done with increasing frequency because, properly executed in a "normal" parturient, it carries only slightly more risk to the mother, and, in the presence of certain complications, it carries less risk to the infant than a difficult vaginal delivery. Optimal results require effective teamwork among obstetricians, anesthesiologists, and nursing personnel: the anesthesiologist should be fully informed of the obstetric aspects; the obstetrician should be well acquainted with anesthetic methods; and the nursing staff has to be aware of both.

BASIC CONSIDERATIONS

There is hardly a serious obstetric complication that cannot be managed by cesarean section with better results than vaginal delivery. Currently, of cesarean procedures being done, 50% are repeat cesarean sections done on an elective basis, while the other 50% are primary cesarean sections that are done either electively or as emergency procedures. Of this latter group, 50% are done for either fetal or maternal dystocia (most commonly, cephalopelvic disproportion, dysfunctional labor, or malpresentation); 20% are done for maternal bleeding; and the remaining 30% are done for fetal distress, toxemia, intercurrent disease, and miscellaneous disorders. Many obstetricians believe that most cases of breech presentation can be delivered more safely with cesarean section than by vaginal delivery. Table 17 lists the common indications for cesarean section.

Physiopathology

Effects on the Mother. Cesarean section imposes on the *normal mother* slightly greater stress from physiologic alterations and increased risks in morbidity and mortality than are associated with uncomplicated vaginal delivery. The magnitude depends upon the indication for abdominal delivery and the state of health of the parturient. In healthy women undergoing elective cesarean section, the major stress is usually limited to cardiovascular and respiratory changes. The blood loss is about 1,000 ml, and there is a slightly greater risk associated with intraabdominal major operation and the required anesthesia than with vaginal delivery. In high risk parturients, in addition to the physiologic stress from cesarean section, there is a significant increase in morbidity and mortality in the recovery stage that is due to infection and/or pulmonary complications. Patients undergoing cesarean section for emergency reasons are exposed to the added risks inherent in the complications that prompted the cesarean section and emergency anesthesia.

The major cardiovascular changes *above those at term* that occur during and immediately after abdominal delivery include increases of 40–45% in cardiac output and 60–65% in stroke volume, and decreases of 10–15% in heart rate and total peripheral resistance, resulting in a blood pressure increase of about 10–15%. The degree of change in maternal hemodynamics after the delivery is influenced by many factors, including: maternal position, apprehension, and pain; oxytocics; coexistent disorders such as dehydration, blood loss, anemia, and acidosis; the type of analgesia-anesthesia used; the use of left uterine displacement; and fluid replacement during cesarean section.

Effects on Fetus and Newborn. Properly accomplished, cesarean section imposes less of a risk on the fetus and newborn than does a complicated vaginal delivery. However, compared with *normal* vaginal delivery, even uncomplicated cesarean section is associated with slightly greater perinatal morbidity. The degree of morbidity is influenced by maturity of the fetus; maternal and obstetric complications; *type* and *duration* of analgesia and anesthesia, and quality of anesthetic care; elective or emergency conditions; and the operative technique. A slightly greater perinatal hypoxia, hypercapnia, and acid-base disturbance is associated with elective cesarean section as compared with normal vaginal delivery birth as demonstrated by Apgar scores, acid-base studies, and higher incidence of low Early Neonatal Neurobehavioral Scores (ENNS). In the presence of obstetric complications, there may be a higher incidence of perinatal mortality and morbidity because of the impairment of uteroplacental blood gas transfer caused by the obstetric disorder. Prematurity increases the incidence of neonatal morbidity.

In regard to anesthesia, it is important to recall that the fetus and newborn will have decreases in umbilical artery oxygen tension, pH, and base excess (metabolic acidosis) consequent to maternal hyperventilation, improperly treated hypotension, and hypoxia and/or hypercapnia due to any cause. (See Chapters 8 and 12.) General anesthesia achieved with large doses of intravenous drugs

TABLE 17. INDICATIONS FOR CESAREAN SECTION

ELECTIVE SECTION	EMERGENCY SECTION
1. Previous cesarean section	1. Abruptio placentae
2. Cephalopelvic disproportion	2. Placenta previa
3. Breech presentation	3. Prolapsed cord
4. Malpresentation	4. Fetal distress from other causes
5. Chronic uteroplacental insufficiency	5. Failure to progress
a. Toxemia	6. Failure of induction
b. Diabetes mellitus	7. Failed forceps
c. Hypertension	8. Tetanic uterine contractions
5. Rh Isoimmunization	

and/or high concentrations of inhalation agents is associated with significant fetal and neonatal depression, as are prolonged general anesthesia and inadequate depths of inhalation anesthesia. It has been amply documented that the longer the duration of general anesthesia the greater the drug-induced depression of the newborn (Table 18). Moreover, noxious stimulation inherent in surgical inci-

TABLE 18. EFFECTS OF DURATION OF ANTEPARTUM GENERAL OR EPIDURAL ANESTHESIA ON CLINICAL CONDITION OF NEWBORN (APGAR SCORES)

GENERAL ANESTHESIA[1]		GENERAL (N₂O-O₂) ANESTHESIA[2]		EPIDURAL ANESTHESIA[3]	
Minutes of Anesthesia	Mean Apgar Score	Minutes of Anesthesia	Percent Apgar Scores 7–10	Minutes of Anesthesia	Percent Apgar Scores 7–10
<10 min	7.7	<5+	88	<20	85
11–20 min	6.8	6–10	74	21–30	93
21 min or more	6.3	11–20	69	31–60	92
		21–30	50	61–120	90
		31–60	36	>120	100

1 Finster, M. and Poppers, P.: Anesthesiology 29:190, 1968

2, 3 Shnider, S. M. and Levinson, G.: *Anesthesia for Obstetrics*, Baltimore, Williams and Wilkins, 1979.

sion in the presence of inadequate depth of inhalation anesthesia as obtains with 50% nitrous oxide in oxygen is associated with a significant increase in maternal arterial blood pressure and plasma norepinephrine and a significant decrease in uterine blood flow. Moreover, a significant number (20–25%) of parturients will be aware of the surgery and birth with subsequent nightmares and other unpleasant experiences. Finally, the longer the interval between the time of incision of the uterus and delivery of the infant the lower the pH and Apgar score of the newborn.

Certain conditions pertaining to anesthesia and surgery decrease or eliminate some of these deleterious effects. Using small doses of induction agents (e.g., 0.4–0.5 mg/kg ketamine combined with 2–3 mg/kg thiopental) and 40% nitrous

TABLE 19. EFFECT OF INCREASING MATERNAL OXYGEN TENSION ON THE OXYGENATION AND RESPIRATION OF THE NEWBORN*

Maternal arterial PO_2 mm Hg	61–100	101–240	241–360	361–520
Umbilical venous PO_2 mm Hg	29	29–31	35–38	41
Umbilical artery PO_2 mm Hg	16	20–21	23–25	26
Time necessary for infants to establish sustained respiration (seconds)	62	33–54	11–27	13
Percent of infants with Apgar score of 6 or less	30%	15–20%	0	0

* Modified from Marx, G. F. and Mateo, C. V.: Can. Anaesth. Soc. J. 18:587, 1971

oxide in oxygen supplemented with 0.5% halothane produces minimal or no effects on the newborn. The addition of 0.5% halothane does not increase maternal blood pressure or plasma norepinephrine but significantly increases uterine blood flow. In addition to the benefit to the fetus and newborn, the halothane virtually eliminates maternal awareness without increasing blood loss from depressed uterine tone. Increasing the maternal arterial oxygen tension to 300 mm Hg or above will increase fetal blood oxygen tension, saturation, and content and is associated with better clinical condition of the newborn (Table 19, Figure 58). The induction of general anesthesia is delayed until the surgical team is in the room ready to operate and the patient has been prepped and draped, and the surgeon should deliver the infant within 3 minutes of the uterine incision. If prolonged operating time is anticipated, it is best to use regional anesthesia because, unlike general anesthesia, prolonged regional anesthesia is not associated with neonatal depression (Table 18). Finally, if any hypotension that develops is promptly treated, there is little or no neonatal depression.

ELECTIVE CESAREAN SECTION

The patient should be admitted to the hospital the day before the operation to allow the anesthetist time to adequately carry out preanesthetic care of the pa-

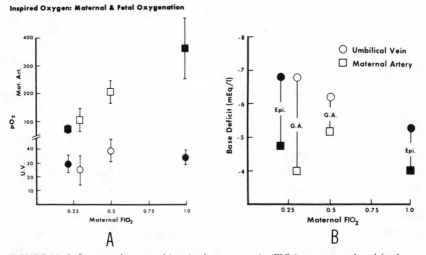

FIGURE 58. Influence of maternal inspired oxygen ratio (FIO_2) on maternal and fetal oxygenation (left) and base deficit (right) at birth by cesarean section. ●■ Epidural analgesia. ○□ Light general anesthesia + relaxant. Fetal oxygenation, acid-base status (and clinical condition) are best when maternal FIO_2 approaches 1.0. (Courtesy of Bromage, P.R.: *Epidural Analgesia*, Philadelphia, W. B. Saunders, 1978. Developed from data of Fox, T. S. and Houle, G. C.: Canad. Anaesth. Soc. J. 18:60, 1971 and Houle, G. C., et al., Anesth. Analg. 48:1011, 1969.)

tient, as discussed on page 64. The anesthetist should be friendly, sympathetic, and use all of his skills to convince the parturient that she is in good hands and that all that can be done will be done for the well-being of herself and the newborn. Since these patients realize that abdominal delivery carries a slightly greater risk and are therefore naturally more apprehensive about the operation and the anesthetic, they require intense psychologic preparation, especially those who are having the operation for the first time. Physical examination is carried out as discussed on page 65. This should include measurement of blood pressure with the gravida on her side and 1, 3, and 5 minutes after she has assumed a supine position. If hypotension develops that is not relieved by lateral displacement of the uterus, regional anesthesia may be inadvisable.

Once the history and physical examinations are completed, the selection of the anesthetic should be discussed with the patient. It deserves emphasis that recent marked advances in knowledge of maternal and perinatal physiology and physiopathology; more sensitive monitoring of the mother, fetus, and newborn; the advent of better anesthetic agents and better understanding of their pharmacology and pharmacokinetics; and, most importantly, the advent of physician anesthetists with a special interest and expertise in obstetric anesthesia have made anesthesia for cesarean section much safer. As a result, provided each method is *properly administered,* there is little difference in maternal and neonatal outcome among the various techniques of anesthesia for elective cesarean section. Therefore, the selection of the optimal anesthetic is based on the following considerations (in order of importance): (a) the knowledge, skill, and experience of the anesthetist with each of the various techniques; (b) the desires of the mother; and (c) the experience of the obstetrician in working with each technique. Assuming that the anesthetist is well-versed with all techniques, then the desires of the other are the primary consideration. If she wishes to be awake, regional anesthesia is selected, whereas, if she expresses fears about having needles in her back or the desire to be asleep, general anesthesia is the choice. Whatever method is selected, the gravida should be reassured and everything done to instill confidence.

Another important part of the preanesthetic preparation is to emphasize to the patient that she sleep on her side and be on her side during her journey from the ward to the operating theater, explaining the reasons for this suggestion. The preanesthetic orders should include: (a) an ample dose of a hypnotic to assure an undisturbed sleep the night before the surgery and (b) a written request for the nurses to be sure that the patient follows the instruction to sleep on her side and be on her side during her journey to the operating theater.

The procedures to be followed during the immediate preanesthetic period are summarized in Table 20. Of special importance are: (a) having the gravida on her side from the time she leaves her room until the induction of anesthesia; (b) re-explaining the anesthetic procedure to the patient and reassuring her repeatedly; (c) starting on intravenous infusion of lactated Ringer's solution with a 16-gauge teflon catheter—if a regional anesthesia is to be used, the solution is

TABLE 20. PREANESTHETIC PREPARATION FOR CESAREAN SECTION

1. Preanesthetic medication 45–60 minutes prior to anesthesia:

   50 mg hydroxyzine IM or chlordiazepoxide (Librium) 20 mg by mouth; avoid narcotics and diazepam because of side effects on the infant

2. 20–30 ml of antacid just before leaving patient's room

3. Transfer patient to operating room in the lateral position

4. Re-explain anesthetic procedure and reassure patient

5. Start intravenous infusion of lactated Ringer's with 16 gauge teflon catheter

   a. If epidural or spinal anesthesia to be given infuse rapidly so that 1,000 ml given by time block established

6. Check and recheck all equipment for anesthesia and *immediate* therapy of complications

   a. Oxygen delivery system and machine for artifical ventilation

   b. Orofacial airway, endotracheal tubes, and laryngoscope

   c. Thiopental/diazepam/succinylcholine solution for immediate injection in case of convulsions

   d. Dilute ephedrine solution (5 mg/ml) for prompt therapy of hypotension

7. Have assistant for psychologic preparation of the parturient and to help anesthetist

---

infused at a rapid rate so that the total volume will have been given by the time the block becomes established; (d) checking and rechecking the equipment for the administration of anesthesia and for the *immediate* therapy of possible complications; and (e) having a well-informed and experienced assistant (usually an obstetric nurse) whose sole responsibility during the entire induction of anesthesia is to provide psychologic support for the patient and to help the anesthetist.

Extradural Block

In recent years, spinal epidural anesthesia achieved with a single injection or by intermittent injection through an indwelling epidural catheter to produce "continuous" analgesia has displaced subarachnoid block as the regional anesthetic of choice for elective cesarean section. This trend has resulted from the advent of better local anesthetics, refinements of the techniques and equipment, and better appreciation of their advantages and limitations. The advantages of spinal epidural analgesia over subarachnoid block for cesarean section are the same as those listed on page 98. These make epidural analgesia more acceptable to the gravida in whom regional anesthesia for cesarean section is desirable but who refuses "spinal" anesthesia. Maternal cardiovascular disturbances are usually less with epidural anesthesia than with subarachnoid block because of the fact that the onset of vasomotor blockade is slower, thus giving the gravida more opportunity to mobilize her compensatory mechanisms. It should be emphasized however that prophylactic measures against aortocaval compression and maternal hypotension are much more important in minimizing the incidence and magnitude of hypotension than the technique used.

In addition to the disadvantages of epidural anesthesia compared with subarachnoid block listed on page 64 related to vaginal delivery, the need to inject a larger dose of local anesthetic to achieve a level of analgesia to T_6 or above theoretically may lead to greater incidence of fetal and neonatal depression manifested by the loss of beat-to-beat variability and lower ENNS. However, recent studies in which the effects of spinal anesthesia achieved with tetracaine were compared with those of epidural analgesia achieved with 0.75% bupivacaine showed no difference in the ENNS scores between the two groups.

The prophylactic measures to prevent maternal hypotension are the same as discussed on page 100, and include an intravenous infusion of 1,000 ml of lactated Ringer's solution administered by the time the block is complete and having the patient lie on her side before and during the induction of epidural anesthesia.

The technique is similar to that described on page 101 for vaginal delivery, except that a larger volume of local anesthesia is used. The epidural puncture is done at the third lumbar interspace using the lack-of-resistance test, and a catheter is then advanced 3-4 cm cephalad, the needle removed, and the catheter fixed in place. After attempts at aspiration, a test dose of 2 ml is injected, and if no evidence of subarachnoid block occurs in 5 minutes, a therapeutic dose of 15–20 ml (depending on the height of the patient) of 0.75% bupivacaine is injected. Some clinicians inject the therapeutic dose in increments of 8–10 ml injected at intervals of 3–4 minutes. Following the injection of the therapeutic dose, some clinicians insist that the patient remain on her side for 3–4 minutes and then turn to the opposite side to prevent unilateral analgesia. Others prefer to inject the therapeutic dose with the patient in the supine position, but with the uterus displaced laterally. In any case, left lateral tilt is used as soon as the parturient assumes the supine position (Figure 59).

Immediately after the injection is completed, the mother should be given supplementary oxygen through nasal prongs or a clear plastic mask, and the blood pressure, pulse, and fetal heart rate are measured and repeated every 30 seconds for the first 10 minutes, and then every minute thereafter until block is established. An automatic noninvasive blood pressure and pulse monitor with an alarm system and a continuous ECG is advisable, especially for all high risk pegnancies. At the first sign of hypotension, a check should be made to ascertain that the uterus is being effeitvely displaced laterally, and, if this is the case and the patient remains hypotensive, she is given increments of 10 mg of ephedrine intravenously, and this is repeated to maintain blood pressure near normal. The anesthetist should remain in close verbal contact with the patient to promptly detect any sign of systemic drug toxicity or total spinal anesthesia.

It deserves emphasis that usually it requires 15–20 minutes for complete anesthesia to develop. The level of analgesia is tested, beginning about 7–8 minutes after the injection of the therapeutic dose, and, if hypalgesia extends to the 6th thoracic dermatome, the preliminary preparation of the skin and draping can

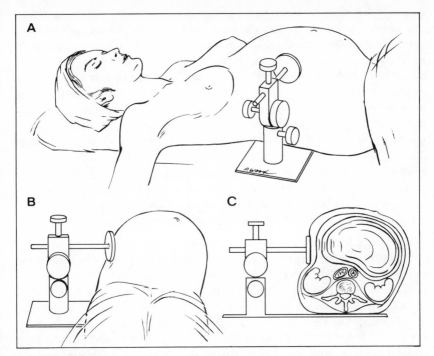

FIGURE 59. Technique of left uterine displacement device (LUDD) with the Colon-Morales apparatus in a parturient about to undergo cesarean section with epidural anesthesia. After induction of epidural block, assumption of the supine position caused the mean arterial pressure to drop from 92 mm Hg to 73 mm Hg, but it was promptly restored to 90 mm Hg as soon as the LUDD was applied. Other circulatory variables during the control (C) period, epidural block (EB), and LUDD were as follows: cardiac output (1/min): 8.9, 6.9, 8.5; total peripheral resistance (dynes/sec/cm^{-5} upper part): 861, 1068, 890.

be initiated. It is essential, of course, that the surgeon not begin the operation until complete anesthesia has been established.

The patient should be given psychologic support throughout the procedure, and, if the parturient manifests undue anxiety in the presence of an adequate level of analgesia, she is given intravenous increments of 2.5 mg of diazepam. If the operative maneuver produces pain, the patient is reassured and given either 40% nitrous oxide in oxygen or 0.25 mg/kg of ketamine intravenously, and after delivery of the infant she is given increments of narcotics as well as continuation of the 40% nitrous oxide in oxygen supplemented with 0.25% methoxyflurane. If the patient experiences severe discomfort because of inadequate anesthesia or is emotionally upset, it is advisable to administer general balanced anesthesia as described below.

Subarachnoid Block

Despite the recent trend of favoring spinal epidural anesthesia for cesarean section, subarachnoid block remains a frequently used method for this purpose. In addition to the advantages common to regional anesthesia, subarachnoid block has the following advantages over spinal epidural anesthesia: (a) simpler technique and lower failure rate; (b) more rapid onset of anesthesia; (c) it requires 1/10 or 1/8 the amount of local anesthetic needed for spinal epidural anesthesia, and consequently there is no risk of maternal systemic toxicity or fetal or neonatal depression. Maternal safety is attested by the fact that hundreds of thousands of patients have been given spinal anesthesia for cesarean section without serious complications. Neonatal benefits of this technique have been demonstrated by statistics from many centers where spinal anesthesia is used extensively by skilled personnel. The greater appreciation of the importance of preventing or minimizing maternal hypotension with uterine displacement, intravenous infusions, and administration of small doses of ephedrine have made spinal anesthesia not only safe but beneficial to the mother and newborn.

Technique. The technique for subarachnoid block is described in Chapter 10, and only a few points pertinent to cesarean section are made here. Dural puncture with a small bore (25 or 26 gauge) needle is done at the 3rd or 4th lumbar interspace. In the average parturient, 7–8 mg of tetracaine diluted with 5% dextrose to a total volume of 2 ml is injected slowly. In smaller, shorter patients the dose is reduced to 6 mg, while in taller patients, it is increased to 9 mg diluted to 2.5 ml. Lidocaine, 37.5 to 50 mg in dextrose, is preferred by some clinicians because it produces more rapid and intense anesthesia. Some clinicians prefer to have the patient on her side during the establishment of the block and have her change sides after 3 minutes to decrease the risk of unilateral analgesia. Others prefer the supine position with effective lateral displacement of the uterus.

The mother is given oxygen, and vital signs are measured as described with epidural block. Three minutes after the subarachnoid injection, the level of hypalgesia and analgesia is determined by pin prick test. The level of analgesia should be made to extend to the 5th–6th thoracic dermatome; if the level is inadequate, the table is tilted 5 ° Trendelenburg and the level checked every 30 seconds until adequate. No attempt should be made to reverse the diffusion of the drug by the reverse Trendelenburg position because this may drastically reduce venous return and can quickly lead to profound hypotension, cerebral ischemia, and even cardiac arrest.

As soon as hypalgesia to the 6th thoracic dermatome develops, the surgical preparation of the abdomen is initiated, and, by the time it is completed, the anesthesia should be adequate for the surgical incision. The management of the patient is the same as described with epidural anesthesia.

Local Infiltration

If an experienced anesthetist is unavailable, local infiltration or field block of the abdominal wall effectively carried out serves admirably for elective cesarean section. Theoretically, this method of anesthesia imposes the least amount of stress and should be the safest method from the point of view of both mother and baby. Unfortunately, it is done so infrequently that most obstetricians have had little or no experience with the technique. Consequently, in the rare case when it is employed, field block anesthesia is often done improperly, and the patient experiences pain during the operation or develops systemic toxic reactions, or both. This technique is not recommended except for those who have had extensive experience with it. To avoid the risk of systemic toxic reactions, it is essential to use very dilute solutions of local anesthetic such as 0.5% 2-chloroprocaine, 0.25% lidocaine or mepivacaine, or 0.05% tetracaine or bupivacaine. These concentrations produce adequate analgesia and permit the use of as much as 150 ml of solution with little or no risk of systemic reactions. However, the onset of anesthesia is slower and it is therefore essential to wait until the drug has had time to produce adequate anesthesia.

Balanced Anesthesia

Recently there has been a progressive increase in the use of balanced anesthesia for cesarean section. The technique is the same as summarized on page 110 and consists of the following sequence. Five minutes before the induction of anesthesia, the gravida is given 100% oxygen at high flows and 3 mg of d-tubocurare or 1 mg of pancuronium intravenously to prevent fasciculation from the subsequent succinylcholine. This is followed by a rapid sequence of: administration of a single dose of 0.5 mg/kg ketamine followed immediately with a single dose of 3 mg/kg of thiopental and then 100 mg of succinylcholine, while cricoid pressure is applied. Once paralysis develops, an endotracheal tube is inserted, the cuff is inflated, and the adequacy of ventilation is ascertained. At this stage, the cricoid pressure is released and the obstetrician is informed that he may proceed. A light plane of inhalation anesthesia is then maintained with 40% nitrous oxide in oxygen supplemented with 0.5% halothane, and muscle relaxation is continued with an intravenous infusion of succinylcholine or single doses of d-tubocurare or pancuronium. The latter relaxants are preferred by many clinicians because they can be reversed at the end of the procedure. The anesthetic is continued until after delivery of the infant, at which time the nitrous oxide can be increased to 60%, the halothane eliminated or decreased to 0.25%, and small increments of narcotics given to assure adequate anesthesia. It is important to avoid maternal hyperventilation for reasons previously given. The patient is extubated when she awakens.

Properly utilized, this technique: (a) results in little effect on the fetus and newborn or the uterus; (b) has no significant alteration in the acid-base status of the mother or neonate; and (c) produces less cardiovascular disturbance than spinal or epidural anesthesia. These advantages, along with rapid, smooth, and pleasant induction and emergence from anesthesia, have made the technique

171

popular among obstetricians, patients, and anesthesiologists. In some centers it has displaced regional anesthesia as a method of anesthesia for cesarean section. Recent studies of the acid-base status and activity of the neonate have shown that balanced anesthesia compares favorably with spinal anesthesia, provided severe hyperventilation of the mother is avoided and the time of induction to delivery of the infant is not more than 10 minutes. Therefore, the induction of anesthesia should be delayed until just prior to the surgical incision.

EMERGENCY CESAREAN SECTION

In selecting anesthesia for emergency cesarean section, consideration must be given to: (a) the degree of urgency; (b) the associated physiopathology; (c) condition of the mother; (d) the condition of the fetus; (e) the skill and experience of the anesthetist; (f) the surgeon's experience and requirements for anesthesia; and (g) the type of analgesia used prior to cesarean section. Although all of these factors are important, the degree of urgency and the skill and experience of the anesthetist are the most critical and determine the method of anesthesia to be utilized.

Dystocia. Emergency cesarean section is often carried out after an unsuccessful trial of labor or trial of forceps in patients with cephalopelvic disproportion or dysfunctional labor. Most of these patients are in good physical condition, well hydrated, and in normal acid-base status; however, they may be physically and emotionally exhausted unless sedatives and narcotics or regional analgesia or self-administered inhalation analgesia have been utilized during labor.

If continuous spinal epidural analgesia has been in use prior to the time a decision is made to proceed with cesarean section, the level of analgesia is extended to the 5th–6th thoracic dermatome by injecting an appropriate volume of 0.75% bupivacaine or, preferably, 1.5% etidocaine because of its shorter latency. If continuous epidural analgesia has not been used during labor, subarachnoid block is the regional anesthetic of choice. In addition to those advantages mentioned previously, spinal anesthesia is especially useful whenever the mother has had large doses of sedatives and narcotics during labor or when there is danger of aspiration of undigested food and fluid.

Balanced anesthesia is the procedure of choice if the other techniques are not practical or are contraindicated. It is also the choice in patients who strongly dislike regional anesthesia or who are otherwise emotionally unsuited for it.

Hemorrhage. Emergency cesarean section in the event of hemorrhage requires optimal teamwork and expert anesthetic care if the mother and infant are to survive. If blood is not available and hemorrhage is very active, the operation must be started as soon as possible, utilizing ample amounts of available volume expanders. Balanced general anesthesia as described above is definitely the best and safest method for mother and infant. Regional anesthesia in any form is contraindicated.

Fetal Distress. In most instances of fetal distress, balanced general anesthesia is indicated because immediate delivery is necessary to save the infant. Even when a continuous epidural catheter is in place, the time necessary to produce surgical anesthesia may be unnecessarily long. Although some clinicians can induce subarachnoid block within 5 minutes, even this may be too long a time before surgical intervention can be carried out.

Tetanic uterine contractions occasionally must be relieved immediately to prevent newborn morbidity or mortality. The most effective way to achieve uterine relaxation is to use balanced anesthesia including halothane. When halothane is administered in a 2% concentration the uterus relaxes within 90–120 seconds, and the condition of the fetus improves. Because of such rapid induction the anesthesia is often associated with moderate cardiovascular depression and hypotension; therefore, the halothane administration should be stopped when the relaxed uterus is exposed. Hyperventilation with nitrous oxide and oxygen eliminates the halothane, and the uterus regains its tone following delivery. Beta adrenergic drugs and magnesium sulphate may also be utilized to relax the uterus; however, these are not as effective as halothane.

CHAPTER 16. MANAGEMENT OF THE NEWBORN (INCLUDING RESUSCITATION)

The neonatal period is the time of greatest mortality in childhood with the highest risk occurring during the first 24 hours of life. Contributing to this are social, economic, genetic, metabolic, physiologic, and iatrogenic factors. These occur during gestation, delivery, and postnatal period and have a major impact on the neonate. At birth, fetal circulation and dependence upon the mother for its well-being cease, and the circulatory and respiratory systems must undergo dramatic changes. Normal neonates undergo these changes with little or no difficulty, and they establish good pulmonary ventilation and cardiovascular function. In the remainder, a variety of causes impair the establishment of adequate respiration and perfusion and necessitate infant resuscitation. This chapter discusses briefly the initial clinical management and resuscitation of the newborn.

BASIC CONSIDERATIONS

Optimal care of the neonate requires adherence to certain principles including: (1) full knowledge of fetal and neonatal physiology and of the medical and obstetric history of the parturient and of the course of labor; (2) a practical and uniform method of evaluating the newborn that will permit any member of the obstetric team to make a prompt diagnosis of neonatal depression; (3) thorough familiarity with measures for the prevention and effective therapy of neonatal depression (and skill in their performance) by every member of the obstetric team; (4) a plan for coordinated teamwork with definite delineation of responsibility for prompt resuscitation under different conditions; and (5) availability of modern resuscitation equipment in good working condition. Moreover, it is the responsibility of the obstetric team to identify the high risk fetuses prior to birth and prepare for immediate resuscitation of the newborn (Table 21).

To avoid repetition, the reader is referred to Chapter 2 for a review of the physiology of the fetus and newborn, especially the respiratory and circulatory changes that occur in the neonate. To state it simply, during the first breath, the undepressed newborn frequently develops a negative intrathoracic pressure of about -45 cm H_2O (range -20 to -70 cm H_2O) causing 40 to 70 cm^3 of air to be drawn in. Then it usually cries and expires against a partially closed glottis which prevents an egress of about 1/2 of the inspired air, with the remainder being left to build up the residual volume. Subsequently, there is a period of transition of irregular breathing after which the pattern becomes regular and the respiratory rate increases to 40–50 breaths per minute (Figures 24 and 25, pp 36, 37).

This ventilation pattern helps the vigorous newborn to recover from birth asphyxia which to some degree occurs during all births. During the first few seconds after birth, the $PaCO_2$ rises sharply but, with the onset of transitional breathing, it falls rapidly and oxygen tension increases (Figure 60a). However,

TABLE 21. SOME FACTORS THAT CAUSE HIGH-RISK PREGNANCIES*

MATERNAL CONDITIONS	Score[+]	FETAL CONDITIONS	Score
Toxemia	10	Prematurity or postmaturity (43 wks)	10
Hypertension	10	Intrauterine growth retardation	10
Heart disease (II-W)	10	Multiple births	10
Diabetes mellitus	10	Hydramnios	10
Chronic renal disease	10	Meconium stained amniotic fluid	10
Maternal infection	10	**LABOR AND DELIVERY CONDITIONS**	
Previous fetal or neonatal deaths	10		
Prolonged ruptured membranes	10	Breech or other abnormal presentation	10
Previous endocrine ablation	10	Prolapsed umbilical cord	10
Uterine or pelvic abnormalities	10	Nuchal cord	10
Maternal malnutrition	8	Uterine rupture	10
Severe obesity	5	Placenta previa or abruptio	10
Pulmonary disease	5	Fetal bradycardia or tachycardia	10
Sickle cell disease	5	Fetal acidosis (pH < 7.25 1st stage)	10
Anemia (< 9 gm Hb)	5	Anesthetic complications (hypotension or hypoxia)	10
Rh sensitization	5		
Third trimester bleeding	5	Forceps delivery	5
Drug or alcohol abuse	5	Cesarean section	5
Elderly (> 35 yrs) or very young (< 15 yrs)	5	Prolonged general anesthesia	5
Epilepsy or thyroid disease	5	Excessive sedation or analgesia	5
		Prolonged or precipitous labor	5
		Uterine hypertonus (spontaneous or oxytocin-induced)	5

* Modified from Hobel, C.J., et al., Am. J. Obstet. Gynecol. 117:1, 1973.

+Numerical scores assigned arbitrarily by authors to reflect degree of risk in relation to neonatal outcome; the higher the score, the greater the risk.

the metabolic acidosis continues to increase for several more minutes but, with the onset of good, regular ventilation, $PaCO_2$ continues to decrease, PaO_2 continues to rise, and recovery from birth asphyxia begins. The rate of recovery is at first rapid, but then proceeds more slowly, and at one to two hours of life, the acid-base state has become stabilized.

Infants who do not ventilate properly immediately after birth will have a slower rate of recovery from birth asphyxia (Figure 60a). Factors that depress ventilation and thus slow the rate of recovery from birth asphyxia include prematurity, analgesics, anesthetics and other depressant drugs, and maternal or obstetric complications that impair uteroplacental blood flow and thus produce more serious birth asphyxia (Table 21). During the immediate postnatal period, a

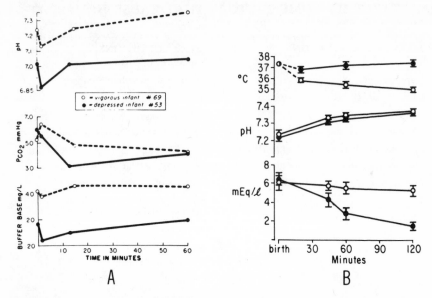

FIGURE 60. *Left:* The pattern of change in pH, CO_2 tension, and buffer base in a vigorous infant (dotted line) compared with that of a severely asphyxiated infant (continuous line). After 3½ minutes of artificial ventilation, the depressed infant took the first deep breath and sustained respiration continued, but it took several hours for restoration of normal acid-base status. Note the initial drop in pH in buffer base and rise in PCO_2 before recovery begins. *Right:* Effect of body temperature on the acid-base state of the newborn. The top curve shows deep body (colonic) temperature and the lowest curve the base deficit during the first 2 hours of life in two groups of healthy infants. In one group body temperatures were mantaned by infrared lamp (●); in the other, (○), body temperatures were allowed to fall while infants were exposed to environmental temperatures at 25° C (room temperature). (Courtesy of James, S.L.: Bull Sloane Hosp. for Women 5:107, 1959.)

fall in pH and buffer base and the rise in $PaCO_2$ and lactate are greater and of longer duration in the depressed infant than they are in the vigorous infant. Whereas, the vigorous infant has recovered to near-normal acid-base state by 1 hour of age, the depressed infant is still moderately to markedly acidotic (Figure 60).

Under conditions of apnea, the oxygen content of arterial blood falls to near zero in 2½ minutes, carbon dioxide tension rises at the rate of about 10 mm Hg a minute, and pH falls about 0.1 pH unit every 3 minutes. As a consequence, there is further depression of the respiratory center, myocardium, and peripheral vascular bed, increased pulmonary vasoconstriction, shunting and atelectasis, loss of muscle tone, and impaired or absent reflex responses. Unless prompt resuscitation is carried out, the central nervous system, as well as other vital organs, are permanently damaged. Therefore, *the practice of some physicians to carry out no active resuscitation in the apneic newborn is to be decried.*

Certain important points are obvious in the proper management of newborn infants. *First,* oxygen is essential for optimal respiratory center performance and to facilitate the circulatory changes. Increasing the oxygen tension of the inspired mixture given to depressed infants increases available oxygen for the increased consumption of the neonate, decreases pulmonary vascular resistance, and improves respiratory performance. *Second,* drastic sensory stimulation by the physician, e.g., spanking, contrast baths, and violent tossing of the infant, sometimes induces gasping or breathing in a depressed infant who is apneic. Drastic sensory stimulation may, however, cause harmful hemodynamic alterations or even result in serious injury to the brain, liver, and viscera. *Third,* prompt controlled or assisted ventilation is the most critical part of resuscitation of the newborn. *Fourth,* adding carbon dioxide to the inspired air (thus further augmenting the level of an already increased blood carbon dioxide) not only is ineffective in improving respiration of the depressed neonate but actually further depresses the infant's respiratory mechanism.

GENERAL MANAGEMENT

The delivery room must be prepared for adequate and prompt treatment of severe neonatal asphyxia. An area designated for neonatal resuscitation close to the site of delivery is mandatory. Every piece of apparatus necessary for emergency resuscitation should be carefully checked as present and functioning before each delivery. All members of the delivery team should be trained and familiar with the methods and equipment necessary for resuscitation. There should be a separate suction apparatus for the newborn, a neonatal oropharyngeal airway, neonatal laryngoscope, several neonatal endotracheal tubes and stylet, a large-bore sterile plastic suction catheter, and a small gauge suction catheter that will traverse the endotracheal tube for suctioning if necessary. Oxygen should be available by means of a bag and mask device and also for insufflation. The resuscitation area should be warmed with some form of radiant heat, and a clearly audible alarm timer should always be utilized to clearly designate 1 and 5 minutes.

Immediate Care

The first step in the care of the newborn is to *establish and maintain a* clear airway. Gentle suction of debris from the oropharynx with a bulb or catheter is done even before delivery of the body. Suctioning of the pharynx and nose should be brief and gentle because prolonged or too vigorous suctioning may produce breath holding, laryngeal inhibition, and even laryngospasm and profound bradycardia. Since gravity is more important in clearing the airway than any mechanical device and in effectiveness is second only to the infant's own cough, the head must be kept lower than the trunk during and immediately after birth until the infant is transported to the resuscitation table (Figure 61). The optimal position on the table is head-down with a slight lateral tilt and the neck extended (Figure 62). Further aspiration of the mouth, pharynx, and nose (in

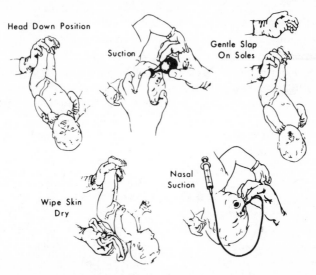

FIGURE 61. Initial management of the newborn consists of establishment of patency of the upper airway by gravity drainage and suction of the pharynx. Once this is completed, a stimulus to cry can be effected by a gentle slap on the soles of the feet or rubbing the infant with a towel. Gentle nasal suction causes the infant to cough and thus to bring up secretions from the trachea to the pharynx. (Courtesy of Gregory, G.A.: *In* Shnider, S.M., and Moya, F. (Eds.): *The Anesthesiologist, Mother and Newborn*, Baltimore, Williams and Wilkins, 1974 pp. 200–209.)

that order) with a catheter is carried out once the infant is on the table, to make sure that all secretions and blood have been removed. It deserves reemphasis that aspiration should be brief and gentle but effective. It is also useful to *gently* apply tactile stimulation to the soles of the feet to help the infant establish rhythmic respirations and provoke crying which is an effective way to bring about the needed changes in lung volumes.

Maintenance of body temperature is one of the most important aspects of the care of the neonate. It is especially important in depressed infants or infants with impaired pulmonary function. The infant should be wrapped *as soon as it* is delivered and then should be dried quickly and placed in a positive thermal environment. Unless this is done, the temperature of the neonate will fall precipitously, resulting in a marked increase in oxygen consumption, metabolic acidosis and respiratory difficulties. The baby should be kept warm by a radiant heater mounted above the bassinet (resuscitator) where the heat source should

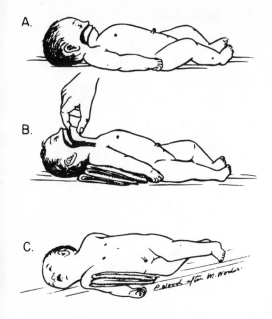

A.

B.

C.

FIGURE 62. Improper (A) and proper (B,C) position of the newborn. In the supine position, the large head forces the lower jaw backward and the tongue blocks the airway, which can be relieved by traction on the lower jaw or placing the infant on the side. (Courtesy of Bonica, J.J.: *Principles and Practice of Obstetric Analgesia and Anesthesia,* Philadelphia, F. A. Davis Company, 1969.)

be servo-controlled by a sensor placed near the baby. If a sensor is not available, a simple infra-red heating lamp may be used, but, precautions must be taken to avoid excessive warming or indeed burning of the infant (Figure 60b).

Clinical Appraisal of the Newborn

Clinical appraisal of the newborn begins with birth. The times of the first gasp, first cry, and the onset of sustained respiration are noted and recorded. The time for sustained respiration (TSR) denotes the time (measured in minutes) following delivery that elapses before the infant begins to maintain a regular and adequate ventilatory activity. If the infant achieves TSR in less than 1 minute, it is recorded as 0.

Apgar Score. The Apgar score at 1, 5, and sometimes at 10 minutes remains the most widely used method to evaluate the clinical condition of the newborn. The five criteria are heart rate, respiratory effort, muscle tone, reflex irritability, and color. The score of 0, 1, or 2 is assigned according to the absence or presence and vigor of each sign (Table 22). A score of 10 represents an infant in the best possible condition and a score of 0 represents a dead infant.. Scores of 1, 2, and 3 indicate an infant in an extremely serious condition.

This scoring system serves as a useful guide to: (1) the need for resuscitation; (2) description of the recovery rate of an infant whose condition was previously active or depressed; and (3) identification of infants at high risk with regard to mortality and morbidity. The 5-minute score is more predictive of survival or

TABLE 22. THE APGAR SCORE

SIGN	Apgar Score		
	0	1	2
Heart rate	Absent	Below 100	Over 100
Respiratory effort	Absent	Slow, irregular	Good crying
Muscle tone	Limp	Some flexion of extremities; poor tone	Active motion
Reflex irritability	No response	Some motion grimace	Cough, sneeze, or cry
Color	Blue, pale	Body pink, extremities blue	Completely pink

neurological abnormality at 1 year of age than the 1-minute score, since the longer asphyxia exists the more likely death or permanent damage will occur.

Because color does not correlate well with the acid-base status of the newborn, J. S. Crawford has recommended that "an Apgar score minus color," or the A-C score, be used at 1, 5, and if necessary, at 10 minutes.. If the $A-C_1$ is 7 or 8, the infant is vigorous; if it is 4–6, it indicates moderate immediate depression; if $A-C_1$ is 3 or less, it indicates severe immediate depression. An $A-C_5$ of 7 indicates moderate, prolonged depression whereas, if it is less than 7, it reflects severe prolonged depression.

Management of Vigorous Neonate

One minute after birth, the majority of infants are breathing well or are crying vigorously and have Apgar scores of 8, 9, or 10. These infants need only the routine newborn measures that are given to all babies. It is preferable to give 100% oxygen for 60 seconds to even vigorous neonates to speed up the increase in oxygen tension and to facilitate the adaptive circulatory changes. This is especially important if the vigorous newborn was delivered of a mother who had received inhalation anesthesia to facilitate its elimination (Figure 63). A brief physical examination for obvious congenital anomalies should also be performed and should include a measurement of blood pressure by Doppler shift sphygmomanometer or similar external device. A normal systolic pressure in a full term newborn is 65–70 mm Hg; a pressure below 50 mm Hg is considered hypotensive.

Within 5 minutes after the infant has established regular ventilation, a nasogastric tube is passed and the stomach is aspirated. This procedure is done to prevent aspiration of gastric contents in the immediate neonatal period and to help in the diagnosis of choanal atresia, esophageal atresia, and small bowel obstruction. The procedure entails passing a soft 8 French plastic catheter attached

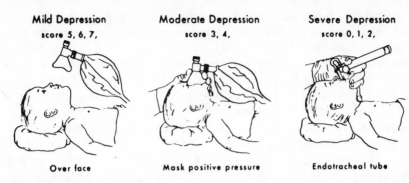

Mild Depression	Moderate Depression	Severe Depression
score 5, 6, 7,	score 3, 4,	score 0, 1, 2,
Over face	Mask positive pressure	Endotracheal tube

FIGURE 63. Techniques of oxygen administration depending upon the clinical condition of the newborn. (Courtesy of Shnider, S.M.: Pediat. Mod. 4:40, 1969.) It is advisable to give oxygen by mask to even vigorous and mildly depressed newborns promptly after establishing a patent airway, in order to increase the rate of arterial oxygen tension and thus facilitate circulatory changes. (See text for details.)

to a syringe through the nose and into the stomach. Its position must be confirmed by injecting 2–3 ml of air while auscultating the left upper abdominal quadrant. The stomach is then aspirated and the contents measured. The average amount is 4–8 ml but larger quantities are frequently found after cesarean section. If 25–50 ml of fluid are present, a small bowel obstruction should be suspected; amounts greater than 50 ml indicate the need for an immediate x-ray examination of the abdomen.

RESUSCITATION OF THE DEPRESSED NEONATE

Mildly Depressed Neonate

The mildly depressed neonate at 1 minute shows cyanosis, has not established regular respiration, and may have only fair muscle tone, so that the total Apgar score is 6 or 7. Such an infant usually requires little more than oxygen and stimulation provided by slapping the soles of the feet. The oxygen should be administered using a small mask and bag system with an oxygen inflow of 2–8 liters per minute. In addition to increasing the concentration of oxygen, this system permits augmentation of every 3rd or 4th inspiratory effort by using slight positive pressure.

Moderately Depressed Neonate

Moderately depressed infants have an Apgar score of 4–6, having lost 1 or 2 for color, respiratory effort, and muscle tone, and often 1 for reflex irritability. They are usually cyanotic or pale, have irregular or no respiration, and have little or no limb movement. The heart rate is usually over 100. Unless these infants are given prompt assisted or controlled ventilation with 100% oxygen, the mild acidosis progresses rapidly, and there is consequent fall in cardiac rate and loss of muscle tone. A small oropharyngeal airway may be helpful in preventing upper airway obstruction by the tongue. Assisted or controlled ventilation using the lowest pressure for the briefest time that will expand the lungs should be used.

Since airway pressures in excess of 30 cm H_2O may rupture the lung unless duration of application is short, it is best to begin by giving 100% oxygen at 25–30 cm H_2O pressure for less than a second. Occasionally, even lower pressures (10–15 cm H_2O) can initiate effective ventilation by stimulating sensitive stretch reflexes in the pulmonary tree. After initial expansion, pressures of 5–15 cm H_2O for 1 second duration are used to provide continuous artificial ventilation.

In addition, the infant is stimulated by *gently* slapping the heels. Although severe noxious stimulation and exposure to cold can break through this moderate depression, they should not be used. Lowering the temperature will inrease the metabolic acidosis, while more vigorous stimulation, e.g., dilation of the anal sphincter and back slapping, may cause serious reflex laryngospasm, hemodynamic alterations, or visceral injury. The heel stimulation can be repeated several times. If these measures effect no improvement in 2 or 3 minutes and the heart rate continues to fall, tracheal intubation should be done.

Severely Depressed Neonates

Severely depressed infants (Apgar score 3 or less) require *immediate and vigorous resuscitation.* These infants are usually apneic, flaccid, pale and respond weakly or not at all to reflex stimulation. Some of them have a heart rate over 100 at birth, but this rapidly decreases so that the total score is 2 or 3. Others are totally unresponsive and have a heart rate below 100, giving a score of 1. In some, the cardiac impulse is hardly discernable or not present at all so that the Apgar score is 0. Frequently, these infants have meconium in the nose, mouth, and pharynx and even in the trachea and over the entire body, indicating severe and prolonged asphyxia in utero. Such infants require vigorous resuscitation immediately after they are delivered. *No time should be lost with halfway measures.*

The most important and most critical step in the resuscitation of the severely depressed infant is intermittent inflation of the lungs with pure oxygen. Tracheal intubation should be accomplished by an expert and the infant ventilated with 100% pure oxygen. (Inexperienced personnel are usually better off utilizing an oropharyngeal airway and positive pressure ventilation with bag and mask.) Depending on the size of the neonate, a size 2.0–3.5 mm (8–14 French) endotracheal tube is chosen and is inserted about 2 cm past the vocal cords. If meconium or debris is observed during exposure of the vocal cords, this should be aspirated via the endotracheal tube.

Following intubation, inflation with 100% oxygen through the tube may initiate ventilation. Although 30–40 ml are required in the first few breaths, the normal tidal volume of the neonate is only 15 ml during quiet breathing. Again, the initial pressures should be just enough to cause the infant's upper chest to rise gently. Following tracheal intubation, immediate diagnosis of the correct placement of the tube must be made. If the tube is in the trachea (and not the esophagus): (1) the upper chest is observed to rise with each inflation; (2) breath sounds are heard in both lung bases and there is less sound over the gastric region; and (3) the clinical condition of the infant improves and heart rate increases to over 100 beats per minute (Figure 64).

Assure Adequate Ventilation

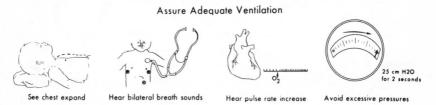

See chest expand   Hear bilateral breath sounds   Hear pulse rate increase   Avoid excessive pressures

FIGURE 64. Means of determining adequacy of ventilation clinically. (Courtesy of Shnider, S.M. (ed.): *Obstetrical Anesthesia, Current Concepts in Practice,* Baltimore, Williams and Wilkins, 1970.)

Meconium-stained Infants

Meconium-stained infants require immediate and, occasionally, vigorous therapy because of the morbidity and mortality associated with its aspiration. Although most infants delivered with but slight meconium staining or amniotic fluid may not be severely depressed or have evidence of aspiration, their airway should be visualized, utilizing a laryngoscope, and the oropharynx and trachea suctioned (along with the nasopharynx) to prevent meconium aspiration into the lung. The depressed infant who is delivered with "tar-like" meconium should have the oropharynx and trachea suctioned immediately, to remove as much meconium as possible, and intubated and suctioned to prevent further aspiration of meconium. Additional therapy is then carried out as described above.

Umbilical Catheterization

In neonates who are unresponsive to therapy and who have Apgar scores of 2 or less at 2 minutes or 5 or less at 5 minutes, umbilical catheterization should be done to measure oxygen tension, acid-base status, and systemic blood pressure and to permit administration of fluids, blood, or appropriate drugs. This procedure requires surgical skill that can only be acquired in the clinical setting. At the same time, gentle cardiac massage is undertaken in the event the severe metabolic acidosis has caused ineffective cardiac action. If the cardiac massage is effective, the infant improves, and the pupils constrict if they were dilated.

Treatment of Acidosis

Fetal or neonatal asphyxia produces respiratory and metabolic acidosis that results in pulmonary vasoconstriction, decrease in surfactant production, and atelectasis. The decreased pulmonary circulation results in continuing neonatal hypoxemia. It is usually easy to correct the respiratory acidosis by ventilation, but severe metabolic acidosis must be corrected with sodium bicarbonate.

The dosage of bicarbonate suggested is 2–5 mEq/kg given at a rate of 1 mEq/kg body weight per minute with or without 10% glucose. In order to provide optimal therapy, a control blood gas should be drawn before and after the bicarbonate administration. Excessive bicarbonate administration is to be avoided to prevent alterations in cardiovascular function and to decrease the hazard of intracranial bleeding. Additional sodium bicarbonate may be administered following a repeat blood sampling and calculation of base excess (deficit). If the base deficit is known, bicarbonate can be calculated by the formula:

$$\text{mEq of NaHCO}_3 = 0.3 \text{ body weight (kg)} \times \text{base excess mEq/L}$$

To avoid the aforementioned hazards, it is advisable initially to attempt to correct half of the residual metabolic component of mixed acidosis and to give the sodium bicarbonate *slowly*.

Fluid Therapy

The normal neonatal blood volume ranges between 70–90 mg/kg. There is an excellent relationship between mean blood pressure and blood volume. Once the umbilical arterial catheter is in place, one can measure mean blood pressure. If the mean blood pressure is below 30 mm Hg in the premature infant or below 40 in the full-term large infant, the infants should receive whole blood but, if this is not available, they should receive an infusion of isotonic saline 5–10 ml/kg body weight over a 2–3 minute period and the response evaluated to determine whether the dose should be repeated immediately. Then salt-poor albumin, 1 gm/kg body weight, should be administered over a 2–5 minute period. An equivalent amount of plasmanate (5–10 ml/kg body weight) may be substituted for the isotonic saline and albumin. Repeated infusions of fluid or whole blood should be given, as needed, to establish and maintain adequate intravascular pressure.

Hypoglycemia should be suspected in infants with intrauterine growth retardation (postmature), or in infants with diabetic mothers, or in infants born fol-

184

lowing severe intrapartum asphyxia. Hypoglycemia is present if the blood sugar is less than 30 mg/100 ml in full-sized infants and less than 20 mg/100 ml in low birth-weight infants and is usually manifested by reduced cardiac output, hypotension, and, when severe, tremors, convulsions, and apnea. It is treated with 5–10 ml/kg body weight of 10% dextrose administered *slowly*. Dehydrated neonates should be given appropriate amounts of fluids and be provided with supplemental sodium administered at a rate of 3 mEq/kg/24 hours, potassium 2 mEq/kg/24 hours after the infant has voided, and calcium 200 mg/kg/24 hours.

Treatment of Cardiac Arrest

If cardiac arrest develops during resuscitation or if no beat is detectable at birth after having been audible through labor, the infant must be quickly suctioned under direct vision and intubated. The lung must be expanded immediately with 100% oxygen. Closed chest cardiac massage is begun with moderate compression of the middle third of the sternum at a rate of 80–100 times per minute (Figure 65). Pressure should be applied to compress the sternum halfway back to

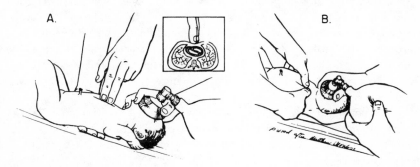

FIGURE 65. Technique of external cardiac massage for cardiac arrest in the newborn. See text for details. (Courtesy of Bonica, J.J.: *Principles and Practice of Obstetric Analgesia and Anesthesia*, Philadelphia, F. A. Davis Company, 1967.)

the vertebral column. Pressure should *not* be applied over the lower third of the sternum, as this maneuver may lacerate the liver. The chest compression should be coordinated with ventilation at a rate of 5 compressions to 1 breath. As previously mentioned, the effect of cardiac massage produces improvement of the neonatal color, constriction of the pupils, and palpable arterial pulses.

If not already done, umbilical vessels should be catheterized and an electrocardiograph applied to monitor heart rate and rhythm. Sodium bicarbonate and 10% dextrose, each in doses of 5 ml/kg, are administered, and, if there is no spontaneous rhythm, epinephrine 10–30 μg (0.1–0.3 ml of a 1:10,000 solution) should be injected into the umbilical vein. Since epinephrine is ineffective in an acidic medium, it should be preceded by the administration of sodium bicarbonate. Calcium chloride in doses of 10–20 mg/kg, administered over a 3–5 minute period may improve myocardial contractility and output. If the heart rate remains below 100 beats per minute, 0.03 mg/kg of atropine or an infusion of dilute solution (16 μg/ml) of isoproterenol should be administered until the heart rate increases and cardiac output improves. The relatively high concentration of isoproterenol is necessary to prevent fluid overload. An alternative method that may be used if the blood volume is adequate is an infusion of dopamine, starting with 5 μg/kg per minute, to increase cardiac output.

Other Drug Therapy

The use of drugs for resuscitation of the depressed neonate should not be considered unless effective ventilation has been initiated. Drug therapy should be conservative and directed towards either temporary support of the failing cardiorespiratory system, counteraction of acidosis, or, when indicated, provision of specific drug antagonists.

If the mother is known to have received narcotics shortly before labor and the neonate manifests signs of narcotic depression (hypoventilation and poor response to stimuli), the infant should be given 100% oxygen using assisted respiration and 10 μg/kg of naloxone (Narcan) should be administered. If the circulation appears normal, the drug is given intramuscularly, but, if circulation is depressed, then a dose of 0.2 μg/kg of naloxone is injected into the umbilical vein or a scalp vein. If the mother is a narcotic addict, the administration of naloxone is contraindicated because the neonate may suffer acute withdrawal symptoms.

Infants born of toxemic mothers who have been treated with large doses of magnesium may display signs of neonatal depression caused by a *magnesium intoxication*. Calcium chloride and calcium gluconate are effective antidotes in this situation.

Newborn infants who are severely depressed with bradycardia, hypotension, apnea, hypotonia, and convulsions should be suspected of local anesthetic toxicity from inadvertent injection of the drug during attempts of caudal or paracervical blocks. Careful examination of the baby's head often discloses the needle puncture site. In addition to the usual resuscitation in the severely depessed neonate, these infants should be detoxified by gastric lavage with isotonic saline and exchange transfusion.

NEUROBEHAVIORAL EVALUATION

More recent data show that the Apgar score used alone is of limited value and helps detect only gross neonatal depression. Consequently, several neurobehavioral methods of evaluating the newborn and the neonatal effects of maternal analgesics have been introduced. At the present time, the most widely used

(Text continues on page 190.)

TABLE 23. EARLY NEONATAL NEUROBEHAVIORAL SCALE (ENNS)*

A. **APGAR SCORE** (total)

B. **STATE** (recorded before each specific test)

Sleep—light sleep (S-1); deep sleep (S-2)

Awake—semi-dozing (A-1); restless (A-2); alert (A-3); intense crying (A-4)

C. **SPECIFIC TESTS**	SCORE			
	0	1	2	3
1. Response to pin prick	Absent	Weak	Brisk	Vigorous
Response decrement to repeated pin prick	Number of stimuli before response alters			
2. Muscle tone evaluations				
Pull to sitting (head control)	Absent	Weak	Shortly erect	Consistently erect
Arm recoil (held to side)	Absent	Weak (45%)	Marked	Strong, overshoot
Truncal tone	Floppy	Weak extension	Vigorous extension	Rigidity
General body tone	Minimal	Weak	Average	Strong
3. Rooting	Absent	Weak	Full head turn	Vigorous
4. Sucking	Absent	1–3 Sucks	3–10 Sucks	Long period sucking
5. Moro's response	Absent	Slow, weak	Moderate, complete	Full, rapid
Response decrement to repeated Moro	Number to alter maximal response			
6. Response decrement to light	Number to alter response			
7. Response to sound	Absent	Slight	Searching	Definite search
8. Placing (standing up of infant)	No response	Minimal flexion	Foot placed	Easy, rapid placing

D. **GENERAL SCORES**

1. Alertness	Dull	Short attentive periods	Long attentive periods	Alert throughout exam
2. Overall assessment	Abnormal	Borderlne	Normal	Superior
3. Predominant state	Recorded as S-1, S-2, A-1, A-2, A-3, A-4			
4. Lability of state	Number of times state changed during exam			

* Modified from Scanlon, J.W. et al.: Anesthesiology 40:121, 1974.

			0	1	2
Adaptive Capacity	1	Response to Sound	absent:	mild:	vigorous:
	2	Habituation to Sound	absent:	7-12 stimuli:	< 6 stimuli:
	3	Response to Light	absent:	mild:	brisk blink or startle:
	4	Habituation to Light	absent:	7-12 stimuli:	< 6 stimuli:
	5	Consolability	absent:	difficult:	easy:

TOTAL [ ] ADAPTIVE CAPACITY

			0	1	2
Passive Tone	6	Scarf Sign	encircles the neck:	elbow slightly passes midline:	elbow does not reach midline:
	7	Recoil of Elbows	absent:	slow; weak:	brisk; reproducible:
	8	Popliteal Angle	>110°	100°-110°	< 90°
	9	Recoil of Lower Limbs	absent:	slow; weak:	brisk; reproducible:
Active Tone	10	Active Contraction of Neck Flexors	absent or abnormal:	difficult:	good; head is maintained in the axis of the body:
	11	Active Contraction of Neck Extensors (from leaning forward position)	absent or abnormal:	difficult:	good; head is maintained in the axis of the body:
	12	Palmar Grasp*	absent:	weak:	excellent; reproducible:
	13	Response to Traction (following palmar grasp)	absent:	Lifts part of the body weight:	lifts all of the body weight:
	14	Supporting Reaction (upright position)	absent:	incomplete; transitory:	Strong; supports all body weight:
*Primary Reflexes	15	Automatic Walking*	absent:	difficult to obtain:	perfect; reproducible:
	16	Moro Reflex*	absent:	weak; incomplete:	perfect; complete:
	17	Sucking*	absent:	weak:	perfect; synchronous with swallowing:
General Assessment	18	Alertness	coma:	lethargy:	normal:
	19	Crying	absent:	weak; high pitched; excessive:	normal:
	20	Motor Activity	absent or grossly excessive:	diminished or mildly excessive:	normal:

TOTAL [ ] NEUROLOGICAL

TOTAL SCORE [ ] AT_____MINUTES OF LIFE

FIGURE 66. Neurologic and adaptive score in full term newborn infants (to be performed any time after 15 minutes of birth).

A. **Adaptive Capacity** (1) *Response to Sound* (RS). Ring bell briskly behind infant's head. If vigorous startle reaction/blinking/respiratory changes, scores RS - **2**; if mediocre - **1**; if absent **0**. (2) *Habituation to Sound* (HTS). After No. (1) ended, repeat sound and note response each time for maximum of 12 times. Score HTS **2** if decrease or change before or at 6th stimulus; if after 7 stimuli, **1**; if no decrease or change - **0**. (3) *Response to Light* (RTL). Briefly shine light into infant's eye and if blinking/startle/eye-widening/motor activity/respiratory change brisk, score RTL **2**; if sluggish/delayed - **1**; if no response - **0**. (4) *Habituation to Light* (HTL). Repeat light stimulus maximum of 12 times and observe sequential reaction. If there is decrease or change in HTL before or at 6th stimulus, score - **2**; if after 7 stimuli - score - **1**; if no response **0**; (5) *Consolability* (C). Measure in infant crying 15 seconds or more. Apply soothing stimulus (examiner's hand on infant's abdomen and restrain activity of upper limbs in prone position and then rock and caress or place finger into mouth). If C rapidly obtained, score - **2**; if obtained with difficulty - 1; if none up to 60 seconds or more - **0**.

B. **Passive Tone** (6) *Scarf Sign* (SS). Holding infant semirecumbent, take hand and pull arm across chest toward opposite shouler to encircle neck like scarf. If elbow does not reach midline (in line with umbilicus), score SS - **2**; if elbow passes midline - **1**; if arm encircles neck without resistance - **0**. (7) *Recoil of Elbows* (RE). With infant supine in flexed posture, pull both hands and fully extend arms; observe how quickly arms flex after release. If brisk, score RE - **2**; if sluggish - **1**; if absent - **0**. (8) *Popliteal Angle* (PA). With infant's pelvis flat on table, flex both thighs on hips and flex knees on sides of abdomen; then lift lower segment of legs and observe leg-thigh angle. If 90° or less, score PA - **2**; if 90–110° - **1**; if more than 110° - **0**. (9) *Recoil of Lower Limbs* (RLL). Infant supine with hips and knees flexed. Extend both legs by pressing on knees and release. If recoil brisk, score RLL - **2**; if sluggish - **1**; if absent - **0**.

C. **Active Tone and Primary Reflexes** (10) *Contraction of Neck Flexors* (CNF). Grasp shoulders and pull supine infant to sitting position and note relation of head to trunk. If head maintained along axis of trunk for 3–5 sec, score CNF - **2**; if head maintained along axis for only 1–2 sec - **1**; if absent or head drops - **0**. (11) *Active Contraction of Neck Flexors* (ACNF). With infant sitting and leaning forward with head hanging on chest, move trunk backward and note reaction of head. If head maintained along trunk axis 3–5 sec, score ACNF - **2**; if maintained only 1–2 sec - **1**; if absent response - **0**. (12) *Palmar Grasp* (PG). Insert examiner's finger into hands from ulnar side and gently press against infant's palm. If infant's grasp strong and reproducible, score PG -**2**; if mediocre - **1**; if absent - **0**. (13) *Response to Traction* (RT). With infant's hands dry, and after eliciting strong palmar grasp, examiner raises index fingers 12 inches (examiner's thumb ready to hold hand and support infant if necessary). If infant flexes upper extremity, lifts body from table and brings feet off table score RT - **2**; if mediocre (i.e., strength of infant's grasp allows only partial body lift) - **1**; if absent - **0**. (14) *Supporting Reaction* (SR). Hold infant by placing examiner's hand on chest and thumb and fingers in axillae. If infant's legs actively straight and trunk muscle contracts to support body weight and maintain position for a few seconds, score SR - **2**; if incomplete and transitory contraction - **1**; if absent response - **0**; (15) *Automatic Walking* (AW). When supporting reaction obtained, automatic walking occurs or is provoked by tilting infant forward. If brisk and reproductible, score AW - **2**; if mediocre (only a few steps taken and not reproduced) - **1**; if absent - **0**. (16) *Moro Reflex* (MR). Hold infant's both hands in abduction while keeping head on bed. Lift shoulder off bed. At maximum passive abduction, release hands briskly. If brisk, active abduction of arms at shoulders, extension of forearms and hands completely open and infant cries, score MR - **2**; if weak or incomplete response (i.e., no crying or hands opening) - **1**; if absent - **0**. (17) *Sucking* (S). Introduce finger into infant's mouth and note strenght and rhythmicity of sucking and synchrony with swallowing. IF S brisk, continuous, and synchronous, give score of **2**; if weak and discontinuous and asynchronous with swallowing - **1**; if absent - **0**.

D. **General Neurologic Assessment** (18) *Alterness* (A). If infant quite alert, eye contact maintained and prompt response to most stimuli, score A - **2**; if lethargic with poor eye contact, short attention span, and sluggish response to stimuli - **1**; if comatose or no response to stimuli - **0**. (19) *Crying* (C). Stimulate to cry and if cry of normal quality/quantity score C - **2**; if abnormal (High pitched, weak, monotonous, discontinuous) - **1**; if no cry - **0**. (20) *Motor Activity* (MA). Observe undistirbed infant. If movements fast, brisk, variable, and harmonious, score MA - **2**; if diminished or excessive motor and unharmonious - **1**; if no MA (i.e., the infant lies motionless and/or when stongly stimulated develops agitation, tremors, or clonic movement) - **0**. After completion of scoring, add scores of each category and total score. Scores above 33–35: condition of infant normal, provided points lost not in one specific category such as tone or adaptive capacity. (Courtesy of Amiel-Tison, C., et al., Anesthesiology, in press.)

method is the Early Neonatal Neurobehavioral Scale (ENNS) developed by Scanlon and associates.. The examination, done at 1 hour after birth and repeated at 4 and 8 hours, consists of several components, as listed in Table 23. The sequence of testing is such as to arouse the infant so that decremental responses will be most accurate and therefore will best reflect behavioral integrity.

An Apgar scoring begins the examination and is meant to serve as an indicator of vital signs. Following this, the general state of the infant is recorded. This is recorded as awake or asleep, and there are degrees of each provided for scoring. The state of the infant is recorded again before each of the specific tests that follow. The specific tests measure the infant's tone, reflexes, and ability to alter behavior in response to noxious or disturbing stimuli. The specific tests include: (1) response to pin prick; (2) muscle tone evaluations; (3) rooting; (4) sucking; (5) Moro's response; (6) response to sound; and (7) placing. Decremental responses include repeated pin prick, Moro, light flash, and sound. Each of these specific tests is scored from 0–3 with the higher number being a more alert, responsive infant. Finally, general scores are added to all the above. These general scores include alertness, overall assessment, predominant state, and lability of state. The ENNS has been proven to have a very high degree of reproducibility among different examiners. The examination is easily taught and fairly quickly administered.

More recently a new method, called ABS (devised by Amiel-Tison, Barrier, and Shnider), has been introduced. It entails neurologic and adaptive capacity scoring and is based on five general areas: (1) adaptive capacity; (2) passive tone; (3) active tone; (4) primary reflexes; and (5) general observations on alertness, cry, and motor activity. Preliminary use of the system has revealed that it is sensitive, easy to learn and carry out, has high interobserver reliability, and correlates well with the ENNS. The developers of the method claim that it has the following advantages over the ENNS: (a) it is learned more quickly and can be completed in 4-5 minutes compared to 7-8 minutes for the ENNS; (b) it places more emphasis on motor tone and therefore is probably more sensitive to drug effect; (c) it avoids noxious stimuli such as pin prick and the repeated Moro maneuvers; and (d) it provides a single number for a given newborn that uniquely identifies a depressed or vigorous neonate. On the basis of these optimistic views, it is reproduced here (Figure 66).

REFERENCES

Abouleish, E.: *Pain Control in Obstetrics*. Philadelphia, J. B. Lippincott, Co., 1977.

Albright, G.A.: *Anesthesia in Obstetrics: Maternal, Fetal, and Neonatal Aspects*. Menlo Park, Addison-Wesley Publishing, Co., 1978.

Amiel-Tison, C., Barrier, B., Shnider, S. M., et al.: A new neurologic and adaptive capacity scoring system for evaluating obstetric medications in full-term newborns. Anesthesiology (in press).

Assali, N. S. and Brinkman, C. R.: The uterine circulation and its control, *in* Longo, L. D. and Bartels, H. (Eds.): *The Respiratory Gas Exchange and Blood Flow in the Placenta*, Bethesda, Maryland; D.H.E.W. Number (NIH) 73–361, 1972, pp. 1-21.

Bonica, J. J.: *Principles and Practice of Obstetric Analgesia and Anesthesia*, Philadelphia, F. A. Davis Company, Vol. 1, 1967, Vol. 2, 1969.

Bonica, J. J.: Maternal respiratory changes during pregnancy and parturition, *in* Marx, G. F. (Ed.): *Parturition and Perinatology*, (Clinical Anesthesia Series), Philadelphia, F. A. Davis Company, 1972.

Bonica, J. J.: Peripheral mechanisms and pathways of parturition pain, *in* Scott, D. B., and Spence, A. A. (Eds.): Proceedings of a Symposium on Current Trends in Obstetric Analgesia, Br. J. Anesth. 51 (Suppl. 1): 3s–9s, 1979.

Bonica, J. J.: Neurophysiologic and pathologic aspects of acute and chronic pain. Arch. Surg. 112:750–781, 1977.

Bromage, P. R.: *Epidural Analgesia*, Philadelphia, W. B. Saunders, 1978.

Caldeyro-Barcia, R. and Poseiro, J. J.: Physiology of the uterine contraction. Clin. Obstet. Gynecol, 3:386–408, 1960.

Covino, B. G. and Vassallo, H. G.: *Local Anesthesia*, New York, Grune & Stratton, 1976.

Chertok, L.: *Psychomatic Methods in Painless Childbirth*. New York, Pergamon Press, 1959.

Crawford, J. S.: *Principles and Practices of Obstetric Anesthesia*, 4th Edition, Oxford, Blackwell Scientific Publications, 1976.

Flowers, C. E., Jr.: *Obstetric Analgesia and Anesthesia*. New York, Harper & Row, Hoeber Medical Division, 1967.

Hytten, F. E. and Leitch, I.: *The Physiology of Human Pregnancy*. Philadelphia, F. A. Davis Company, 1964.

Kerr, M. G., Scott, D. B. and Samuel, E.: Studies of the inferior vena cava in late pregnancy. Br. Med. J., i:532–533, 1964.

Longo, L. D. and Bartels, H. (Eds.): *Respiratory Gas Exchange and Blood Flow in the Placenta*. Bethesda, Maryland, D.H.E.W. Number (NIH) 73–361, 1972.

Marx, G. F. (Ed.): *Recent Research in Obstetric Analgesia-Anesthesia: Clinical Implications*. (Clinical Anesthesia Series). Philadelphia, F. A. Davis Company, 1972.

Marx, G. F. (Ed.): *Clinical Management of Mother and Newborn*. Heidelberg, Springer-Verlag, 1979.

Marx, G. F. and Bassell, G. M. (Eds.): *Obstetric Analgesia and Anesthesia* (Monographs in Anaesthesiology Series Vol. 7). Amsterdam, Excerpta Medica, 1980.

Marx, G. F. and Orkin, L. R.: *Physiology of Obstetric Anesthesia*. Springfield, Charles C. Thomas, 1969.

Moir, D. D.: *Pain Relief in Labour*, 2nd Edition, Edinburgh and London, Churchill Livingstone, 1971.

Moore, D. C.: *Anesthetic Techniques for Obstetrical Anesthesia and Analgesia*. Springfield, Charles C. Thomas, 1964.

Prowse, C. M. and Gaensler, E. A.: Respiratory and acid-base changes during pregnancy. Anesthesiology 26:381–392, 1965.

Ralston, D. H. and Shnider, S. M.: The fetal and neonatal effects of regional anesthesia in obstetrics. Anesthesiology 48:34–64, 1978.

Scanlon, J. W.: Clinical neonatal neurobehavioral assessment: methods and significance, *in* Marx, G. F. (Ed.): *Clinical Management of Mother and Newborn*. Heidelberg, Springer-Verlag, 1979.

Scott, D. B. and Hunter, A. R. (Eds.): Symposium on Obstetric Anesthesia and Analgesia. Br. J. Anaesth. 43:824–902, 1971.

Scott, D. B. and Spence, A. A. (Eds.): Proceedings of the Symposium on Current Trends in Obstetric Analgesia. Br. J. Anaesth. 21 (Suppl. 1), 1979.

Shnider, S. M.: *Obstetrical Anesthesia: Current Concepts and Practice*. Baltimore, Williams and Wilkins, 1970.

Shnider, S. M. and Levinson, G.: *Anesthesia for Obstetrics*. Baltimore, Williams and Wilkins, 1979.

Shnider, S. M. and Moya, F. (Eds.): *The Anesthesiologist, Mother, and Newborn* (9th Postgraduate Seminar in Anesthesiology 1972), Baltimore, Williams and Wilkins, 1973.

Zador, G.: Continuous peridural analgesia and pudendal block for vaginal delivery. (Thesis) Acta Universitatis Uppsaliensis, 184:1–64, 1974.